OCULAR DISORDERS PROVEN OR SUSPECTED TO BE HEREDITARY IN DOGS

American College of Veterinary Ophthalmologists
1992

Prepared for the
American College of Veterinary Ophthalmologists
by the
ACVO Genetics Committee

Dr. Randall H. Scagliotti
Chairman
Carmichael, CA

Dr. Gustavo D. Aguirre
Ithaca, NY

Dr. Cynthia Cook
San Mateo, CA

Dr. Paul F. Dice II
Seattle, WA

Dr. M. Kohle Herrmann
Houston, TX

Dr. Waldo F. Keller
East Lansing, MI

Dr. Denise Lindley
West Lafayette, IN

Dr. Robert J. Munger
Dallas, TX

Dr. Joyce Murphy
Anchorage, AK

Dr. Mark P. Nasisse
Raleigh, NC

Dr. Charles J. Parshall
Richfield Village, OH

Dr. Robert L. Peiffer, Jr.
Chapel Hill, NC

Dr. Gretchen Schmidt
Wheeling, IL

Dr. Cynthia Wheeler
Laingsburg, MI

Compiled by Dr. Mary B. Glaze, Baton Rouge, LA

ERRATA

Dr. David Covitz
Past Chairman
White Plains, NY

Cover illustration: Corey Wheeler

ISBN 0-9635163-0-2

Table of Contents

Forward

The subject matter recorded in this book has been a topic of intense dialogue by members of the American College of Veterinary Ophthalmologists from this college's earliest years. Its development spans a six year period of collective effort on the part of the ACVO Genetics Committee. Advancement in our understanding of veterinary ophthalmic diseases in general, and of veterinary hereditary eye diseases in particular, provided the foundation from which this book has now become a reality. To be sure, the work embodied here represents, in part, fact based on hard data, compromise where the existing data are inconclusive or incomplete, and consensus on the part of the ACVO Genetics Committee in those instances where data are non-existent. With that said, the title, OCULAR DISORDERS PROVEN OR SUSPECTED TO BE HEREDITARY IN DOGS, is intended to imply the dynamic, ever changing nature in which the material in this book should be viewed. In time, through continued research efforts on canine hereditary ocular disorders and from field information derived from the data now accumulating at the newly reorganized Canine Eye Registration Foundation (CERF), some of what we believe to be true today will change. This will result in some ocular diseases gaining addition to the book because they are heritable to certain breeds, while other breeds may have diseases deleted because they are not. As a primer of inherited ocular disorders, this book hopefully will change as the collective effort of students of ocular disease acquire more precise technologies to study the canine genome and its effect on canine ocular health.

Randall H. Scagliotti DVM, MS
Diplomate, ACVO
Chair, ACVO Genetics Committee 1992

Introduction

Although there are noteworthy exceptions, most of the ocular diseases of dogs which are presumed to be hereditary have not been adequately documented. The main reasons for this are:

* related animals are not always available for examination
* controlled breeding trials often impose an economic burden.

The situation is even more difficult when an entity is not present at birth or in the early postnatal period. If an ocular disorder manifests clinically at a later age, it is often impossible to examine an adequate number of closely-related animals. The cost of maintaining a breeding colony for an extended time is often beyond the financial scope of our teaching and research institutions.

Until the genetic basis of an ocular disorder is defined, we must satisfy ourselves with informed opinions and terms like "probably hereditary" and "suspected to be hereditary".

When do we suspect that an entity is inherited?

* when the frequency is greater than in other breeds
* when the frequency increases in a given breed
* when the frequency in a subpopulation of dogs that are interrelated is greater than that noted in unrelated dogs
* when it has a characteristic appearance and location
* when it has a characteristic age of onset and a predictable course (predictable stages of development and time for each stage to develop)
* when it looks identical to an entity which has been proven to be hereditary in another breed

The Genetics Committee of the American College of Veterinary Ophthalmologists (ACVO) is engaged in an ongoing project to update information on ocular disorders proven or suspected to be hereditary in dogs. This compendium is developed based upon published reports, data derived from registry organizations and the experience of the Genetics Committee. In particular, we would like to acknowledge the contribution of The Canine Eye Registration Foundation (CERF) in providing statistical summaries of ophthalmic examinations from their files. The ocular disorders and breeding recommendations which follow are interim guidelines. They will be revised whenever additional evidence becomes available.

It bears emphasizing that the sensitivity of genetic disorder detection is greater when large numbers of dogs are examined. The large number of disorders in this book for some breeds may reflect the popularity of the breed and the numbers of animals evaluated. Conversely, the lack of disorders listed for other breeds often reflects only the paucity of examinations reported. For these reasons the ACVO Genetics Committee strongly recommends annual evaluations of dogs of all breeds as the imperative first step in the control of hereditary ocular disorders.

In this book, we chose the term "BREEDING ADVICE" and purposefully avoided the words "certifiable" and "registerable". To certify, as defined by Webster, is to attest authoritatively, to verify or to testify in writing. ACVO diplomates certify their diagnoses and opinions when they sign an examination form but the ACVO does not serve as a registry. Animal registry organizations may request that the ACVO provide a scientific advisory panel to guide them as they define their guidelines regarding ocular disorders of major concern to each breed. The Genetics Committee is the ACVO's response to such requests. Any national or international registry organization may use diagnoses made by ACVO diplomates in the registering of animals with regard to breeding suitability.

Gonioscopy, tonometry, Schirmer tear testing and electroretinography are not routinely performed during eye screening examinations; thus, dogs with goniodysgenesis, glaucoma, keratoconjunctivitis sicca or some early cases of progressive retinal atrophy might not be detected.

These diagnoses refer only to the **phenotype** (clinical appearance) of an animal. Thus it is possible for a clinically normal animal to be a carrier (abnormal **genotype**) of genetic abnormalities.

The members of the Genetics Committee represent the ACVO but acknowledge that the information generated for a breed may not agree with the knowledge, experience and feeling of every individual ACVO diplomate.

Guidelines Used by the ACVO Genetics Committee in Breeding Recommendations

For each breed, specific ocular disorders have been listed which are known or suspected to be inherited. Two categories of advice regarding breeding have been established:

* **"NO"**: Substantial evidence exists to support the heritability of this entity AND/OR the entity represents a potential compromise of vision or other ocular function.

* **"BREEDER'S OPTION"**: Entity is known or suspected to be inherited but does not represent potential compromise of vision or other ocular function.

When the breeding advice is **"NO"**, even a minor clinical form of the entity would make this animal unsuitable for breeding. When the advice is **"BREEDER'S OPTION"**, caution is advised; in time, it may be appropriate to modify this stand to **"NO"** based on accumulated evidence. If, in time, it becomes apparent that there is insufficient evidence that an entity is inherited, it may be deleted.

An individual ACVO diplomate may disagree with the breeding advice from the Genetics Committee. It is appropriate for this examiner to contact the ACVO Genetics Committee to voice disagreement, initiate change or suggest additions.

There are currently four disorders for which the recommendations against breeding is the same for all breeds:

1. Progressive Retinal Atrophy (PRA): breeding is not advised for any animal demonstrating bilaterally symmetric retinal degeneration (considered to be PRA unless proven otherwise).

2. Cataract: Breeding is not recommended for any animal demonstrating partial or complete opacity of the lens or its capsule **unless the examiner has also checked the space for "significance of above cataract is unknown"**. The prudent approach is to assume cataracts to be hereditary except in cases specifically known to be associated with trauma, other causes of ocular inflammation, specific metabolic diseases, persistent pupillary membrane, persistent hyaloid or nutritional deficiencies.

3. Retinal dysplasia - **geographic or detached**: breeding is not advised for any animal exhibiting a congenital retinal disorder consistent with retinal dysplasia.

4. Retinal detachment: Breeding is not recommended for any animal exhibiting retinal detachment.

Glossary of Terms

Agenesis, Aplasia - failure of development

Anterior - denotes the front portion; e.g. the cornea is **anterior** to the lens.

Anterior chamber - space between the cornea and iris, filled with aqueous humor.

Axis - along an imaginary line connecting the center of the cornea and the retina, **axial** (adj.)

Bilateral - affecting both eyes.

Blepharospasm - squinting; spastic closure of the lids, usually due to pain.

Canthus - junction of the upper and lower lid; one each medial and lateral

Caruncle - fleshy conjunctival tissue at the nasal canthus; may contain hair (**ciliated caruncle**) which, if contacting the cornea, may cause irritation and/or tearing.

Cataract - Lens opacity which may affect one or both eyes and may involve the lens partially or completely. In cases where cataracts are complete and affect both eyes, blindness results. The prudent approach is to assume cataracts to be hereditary except in cases known to be associated with trauma, other causes of ocular inflammation, specific metabolic diseases, persistent pupillary membrane, persistent hyaloid or nutritional deficiencies.

Central Progressive Retinal Atrophy (CPRA) - a progressive retinal degeneration in which photoreceptor death occurs secondary to disease of the underlying pigment epithelium. Progression is slow and some animals never lose vision. CPRA occurs in England, but is uncommon elsewhere.

Choroid - Thin vascular layer that lies between the sclera and retina in the posterior part of the eye.

Choroidal Hypoplasia - an inadequate development of the choroid present at birth. It does not progress as the dog ages.

Chronic Superficial Keratitis - see **Pannus**.

Ciliated caruncle - see **Caruncle**.

Collie Eye Anomaly - a congenital syndrome of ocular anomalies seen in the collie and which includes **choroidal hypoplasia, staphyloma, coloboma**.

Coloboma - a congenital cleft or defect.

Congenital - present at birth. A congenital lesion which may or may not be inherited -- for example an anomaly associated with arrested development due to exposure to a viral infection while in the uterus.

Corneal dystrophy - A non-inflammatory corneal opacity (white to gray) present in one or more of the corneal layers; usually inherited and bilateral.

Dermoid - a patch of skin, usually located on the cornea; its presence usually causes ocular irritation.

Descemet's membrane - the elastic membrane within the deep cornea.

Distichiasis - eyelashes abnormally located in the eyelid margin which may cause ocular irritation. Distichiasis may occur at any time in the life of a dog. It is difficult to make a strong recommendation with regard to breeding dogs with this entity. The hereditary basis has not been established, although it seems probable due to the high incidence in some breeds. Reducing the incidence is a logical goal. When diagnosed, distichiasis should be recorded; breeding discretion is advised.

Dominant - describes the mode of hereditary transmission such that only one of the two genes of a pair must be affected in order for the individual to demonstrate the characteristic controlled by that gene.

> **Incomplete penetrance** - transmission of trait to progeny will result in presence of gene but not its expression.
> **Incompletely dominant** - phenotype differs between heterozygote and homozygote with respect to the gene in question.

Dorsal - upper region; e.g. the upper eyelid is **dorsal** to the lower eyelid (=**superior**).

Dry eye - an abnormality of the tear film, most commonly a deficiency of the aqueous portion, although the mucin and/or lipid layers may be affected; results in ocular irritation and/or vision impairment.

Dysplasia - abnormal development or growth.

Dystrophy - noninflammatory, developmental, nutritional or metabolic abnormality; dystrophy implies a possible hereditary basis and is usually bilateral.

Ectasia - thinning.

Ectopic cilia - hair emerging through the eyelid conjunctiva. Ectopic cilia occur more frequently in younger dogs and cause discomfort and corneal disease.

Ectropion - a conformational defect resulting in eversion of the eyelids, which may cause ocular irritation due to exposure. It is likely that ectropion is influenced by several genes (polygenic), defining the skin and other structures which make up the eyelids, the amount and weight of the skin covering the head and face, the orbital contents and the conformation of the skull.

Ectropion with macroblepharon - Ectropion associated with an exceptionally large eyelid opening and laxity of the canthus structures. Central lower lid ectropion is often associated with entropion of the adjacent lid. This causes severe ocular irritation.

Electroretinogram - a test of retinal function; a graphic record of the electrical response that follows stimulation of the retina by light.

Endothelium (of the cornea) - the most posterior or innermost layer of the cornea.

Entropion - a conformational defect resulting in "in-rolling" of one or more of the eyelids which may cause ocular irritation. It is likely that entropion is influenced by several genes (polygenic), defining the skin and other structures which make up the eyelids, the amount and weight of the skin covering the head and face, the orbital contents and the conformation of the skull.

Epithelium (of the cornea) - the most anterior or outermost layer of the cornea.

Eversion of the cartilage of the third eyelid - a scroll-like curling of the cartilage of the third eyelid, usually everting the margin. The condition may occur in one or both eyes and may cause mild ocular irritation.

Exophthalmos - protrusion of the eyeball; may result secondarily in failure to blink normally and exposure of the cornea (exposure keratopathy syndrome).

Exposure keratopathy syndrome - a corneal disease involving all or part of the cornea, resulting from inadequate blinking. This results from a combination of anatomic features including shallow orbits, exophthalmos, macroblepharon, and lagophthalmos.

Expressivity - the degree to which a given gene manifests itself in the hereditary characteristic which it governs.

Fundus - the posterior portion of the interior of the eye as viewed with an ophthalmoscope; **fundic,** adj.

Genotype - genetic makeup.

Glaucoma - an elevation of intraocular pressure (IOP) which, when sustained, causes intraocular damage resulting in blindness. The elevated IOP occurs because the fluid cannot leave through the iridocorneal angle. Diagnosis and classification of glaucoma requires measurement of IOP (tonometry) and examination of the iridocorneal angle (gonioscopy). Neither of these tests are part of a routine breed eye screening exam.

Goniodysgenesis - a congenital anomaly characterized by the persistence of a sheet of tissue between the base of the iris and the inner corneoscleral junction in the area where drainage normally occurs.

Gonioscopy - a specialized procedure which uses a contact lens to examine the iridocorneal angle.

Hereditary - genetically transmitted or transmissible as a physical characteristic from parent to offspring.

Heterozygote - an individual in which the members of a given pair of genes are dissimilar; **heterozygous**, adj.

Homozygote - an individual in which the members of a given pair of genes are alike; **homozygous**, adj.

Hypoplasia - defective development of an organ or part resulting in a smaller than normal size or an immature state.

Immune-mediated disease - a state in which the immune responses which are essential to the protection of the body act in an unregulated fashion and cause damage.

Imperforate lacrimal punctum - a developmental anomaly resulting in failure of opening of the lacrimal duct adjacent to the eye. The lower punctum is more frequently affected. This defect usually results in epiphora, an overflow of tears onto the face.

Incidence - the rate or range of occurrence; the amount or extent of occurrence; the liability to happen.

Incidental - a chance occurrence; minor; of secondary importance.

Inferior - lower region; e.g. the lower lid is **inferior** to the upper lid (=**ventral**).

Inflammation - redness, swelling, and pain that may or may not be associated with infection.

Intraocular pressure (IOP) - the pressure formed by a balance between intraocular fluid production and outflow.

Iridocorneal angle - the junction between the iris and the cornea; the drainage angle. Aqueous humor leaves the anterior chamber via the trabecular meshwork within the iridocorneal angle into the venous circulation.

Iris - the visible, colored portion of the vascular tunic of the eye, situated in front of the lens, with a central opening, the pupil.

Iris coloboma - a developmental anomaly in which a portion of the iris is absent. It may be a separate disorder or associated with other ocular malformations.

Iris cyst - pigmented cysts arise from posterior pigmented epithelial cells of the iris and remain attached or break free, floating as pigmented spheres of various sizes and pigments in the anterior chamber. Some cysts tend to adhere to the posterior surface of the cornea. Rarely, cysts may be numerous enough to impair vision. The mode of inheritance is unknown.

Iris sheets - continuous layer of uveal tissue bridging the pupil.

Keratitis - inflammation of the cornea; may or may not be associated with infection.

Keratoconjunctivitis sicca (KCS, "dry eye") - inflammation of the cornea and conjunctiva resulting from inadequate aqueous tear production.

Keratoconus - thinning and cone-shaped protrusion of the cornea.

Lagophthalmos - failure to close the eyelids completely; results in exposure of the cornea and conjunctiva.

Lenticonus - an anomaly of the lens in which the anterior or posterior surface protrudes in a conical form; usually congenital.

Limbus - the junction between the cornea and the sclera.

Luxated lens - Partial (subluxated) or complete displacement of the lens from the normal anatomic site behind the pupil. Lens luxation not associated with trauma or inflammation is presumed to be inherited. Lens luxation may result in elevated intraocular pressure (glaucoma) causing vision impairment or blindness.

Macroblepharon - abnormally large eyelid opening; may lead to secondary conditions associated with corneal exposure.

Micropapilla - a small optic disc which is not associated with vision impairment. May be unable to differentiate from **optic nerve hypoplasia** on a routine (dilated) screening ophthalmoscopic exam.

Microphakia - a developmental anomaly present at birth in which there is an abnormally small lens.

Microphthalmia - a developmental anomaly in which the eyeball is abnormally small. This is often associated with other ocular malformations, including defects of the cornea, anterior chamber, lens and/or retina.

Nasal - the region of the eye located toward the nose (**medial**).

Nictitating membrane - third eyelid (haw).

Non-tapetal fundus (non-tapetum) - the area of the fundus which completely surrounds the tapetum.

O.D. - oculus dexter; the right eye.

Optic disc (optic disk; optic papilla) - the part of the optic nerve which is visible in the fundus.

Optic nerve coloboma - a congenital cavity in the optic nerve which, if large, may cause blindness or visual impairment.

Optic nerve hypoplasia - a congenital defect of the optic nerve which causes blindness and abnormal pupil response in the affected eye. May be unable to differentiate from micropapilla on a routine (dilated) screening ophthalmoscopic exam.

O.S. - oculus sinister; the left eye.

O.U. - oculi uterque; both eyes.

Palpebral - associated with the eyelids.

Pannus / chronic superficial keratitis - a bilateral disease of the cornea which usually starts as a grayish haze to the ventral or ventrolateral cornea, followed by the formation of a vascularized subepithelial growth that begins to spread toward the central cornea; pigmentation follows the vascularization. If severe, visual impairment occurs.

Paracentral - situated near the center.

Paraxial - situated along the visual axis.

Persistent hyaloid artery (PHA) - a congenital defect resulting from abnormalities in the development and regression of the hyaloid artery. The blood vessel can be present in the vitreous body as a small vascular strand (PHA) or as a non-vascularized strand that appears gray-white (persistent hyaloid remnant).

Persistent hyperplastic primary vitreous (PHPV) - a congenital defect resulting from abnormalities in the development and regression of the hyaloid artery (the primary vitreous) and the interaction of this blood vessel with the posterior lens capsule/cortex during embryogenesis. This condition is often associated with **persistent tunica vasculosa lentis (PTVL)** which results from failure of regression of the embryologic vascular network which surrounds the developing lens.

Persistent pupillary membranes (PPM) - persistent blood vessel remnants in the anterior chamber of the eye which fail to regress normally in the neonatal period. These strands may bridge from iris to iris, iris to cornea, iris to lens, or form sheets of tissue in the anterior chamber. The last three forms pose the greatest threat to vision and when severe, vision impairment or blindness may occur.

Phenotype - physical appearance.

Pigmentary uveitis - a unique uveitis observed in the Golden retriever, unassociated with other ocular or systemic disorders.

Pole - either extreme of the axis; usually applied to the anterior or posterior axial surfaces of the lens; **polar**, adj.

Prevalence - the percent of a population affected with a disorder at any given time.

Prolapse of the gland of the third eyelid - protrusion of the tear gland associated with the third eyelid. The mode of inheritance of this disorder is unknown. The exposed gland may become irritated. Commonly referred to as "cherry eye".

Progressive Retinal Atrophy (PRA) - a degenerative disease of the retinal visual cells which progresses to blindness. This abnormality may be detected by electroretinogram before it is apparent clinically. In all breeds studied to date, PRA is recessively inherited.

Punctum - one of the two small openings at the nasal eyelid margin which drain the tears away from the eye and into the nasolacrimal drainage system. Abnormalities in the puncta may result in epiphora, or overflow of tears.

Recessive - mode of inheritance in which both genes must be present in order for the characteristic to be expressed in an individual. For a recessive disease, both genes must be abnormal for the disease to be present.

Retinal detachment - the separation of the sensory retina from the underlying tissue. It results in blindness when complete.

Retinal dysplasia - abnormal development of the retina present at birth and recognized to have three forms:

> Retinal dysplasia - **folds**: linear, triangular, curved or curvilinear foci of retinal folding that may be single or multiple.

> Retinal dysplasia - **geographic**: any irregularly shaped area of abnormal retinal development, representing changes not accountable by simple folding.

> Retinal dysplasia - **detachment**: either of the above described forms of retinal dysplasia associated with separation (detachment) of the retina.

The two latter forms are associated with vision impairment or blindness. Retinal dysplasia is known to be inherited in many breeds. The genetic relationship between the three forms of the disease is not known for all breeds.

Schirmer tear test - a test to measure tear production. This test is not part of the routine screening examination.

Sclera - the white, opaque outermost layer of the eyeball.

Sclero-uveitis - an inflammatory disease of the sclera and uvea; the condition may be serious enough to cause blindness.

Staphyloma - an area of corneal or scleral thinning lined by uveal tissue.

Stroma (corneal) - layer of the cornea located between the epithelium and Descemet's membrane; comprises 90% of the corneal thickness.

Subcapsular (lens) - directly under the lens capsule.

Subepithelial (corneal) - directly under the epithelial layer.

Superior - upper region; e.g. the upper eyelid is **superior** to the lower eyelid (= **dorsal**).

Tapetum - the reflective layer in the superior (dorsal) half of the choroid responsible for the shining of an animal's eyes in the dark; this layer may be absent in some animals.

Temporal - the region of the eye located toward the ear (**lateral**).

Tonometry - measurement of the intraocular pressure.

Tunica vasculosa lentis - an embryonic vascularized network which surrounds the lens; the anterior part is the pupillary membrane (see PHPV/PTVL).

Uveal tract (uvea) - the pigmented, vascular layer of the eye comprising the iris, ciliary body and choroid.

Uveitis - inflammation of the uveal tract (iris, ciliary body, choroid). May be caused by infectious agents or may be immune-mediated. There are syndromes of immune-mediated uveitis associated with facial skin depigmentation. Adhesions may develop between the iris and lens (posterior synechia) and the peripheral iris and cornea (peripheral anterior synechia). Other complications include secondary cataract and glaucoma.

Ventral - lower region; e.g. the lower lid is ventral to the upper lid (= **inferior**).

Vesicular - composed of small blisters or bullae.

Vitreal degeneration - a liquefaction of the vitreous gel which may predispose to retinal detachment.

Y sutures (lens sutures) - the y-shaped junction of the lens fibers at the poles. The anterior lens suture is an upright Y; the posterior lens suture is inverted.

Breeds Excluded for Insufficient Data

To date, there are no published reports of inherited ocular conditions in these breeds. In addition, the numbers of individuals for which examinations are recorded are too low to identify the presence of significant ocular disorders.

Affenpinscher
Akbash Dog
American Bulldog
American Eskimo (Spitz)
American Foxhound
American Pit Bull Terrier
American Toy Fox Terrier
Australian Terrier
Azawakh
Belgian Sheepdog - Leaken
Boykin Spaniel
Canaan Dog
Canadian Eskimo
Catahoula Leopard Dog
Chinese Crested
Chinook Husky
Dogo Argentino
Dogue De Bordeaux
Drever
English Foxhound
Entlebuch
Finnish Spitz
Finnish Lapphound
Fila Brasileiro
French Spaniel
German Longhaired Pointer
German Pinscher

Greater Swiss Mountain Hound
Harrier
Kai Ken
Karelian Bear Dog
Kyi Apso
Lakeland Terrier
Leonburger
Mexican Hairless Dog
Norfolk Terrier
Norwegian Buhund
Norwegian Lundhund
Norwich Terrier
Otterhound
Peruvian Inea Orchid Hairless
Petite Basset Griffon Vendeen
Pharaoh Hound
Polski Owczarek Nizinny
Pudelpointer
Scottish Deerhound
Shiba Inu
Skye Terrier
Tahltan Bear Dog
Telomian
Tibetan Mastiff
Tibetan Spaniel
Wirehaired Pointing Griffon

AFGHAN HOUND

	DISORDER	INHERITANCE	REFERENCE	BREEDING ADVICE
A.	Corneal dystrophy	Not defined	1	Breeder option
B.	Cataract	Not defined	2,3	NO

Description and Comments

A.   Corneal Dystrophy

A non-inflammatory corneal opacity (white to gray) present in one or more of the corneal layers. Corneal dystrophy implies a probable inherited basis and is usually bilateral.

B.   Cataract

Lens opacity which may affect one or both eyes and may involve the lens partially or completely. In cases where cataracts are complete and affect both eyes, blindness results. The prudent approach is to assume cataracts to be hereditary except in cases known to be associated with trauma, other causes of ocular inflammation, specific metabolic diseases, persistent pupillary membranes, persistent hyaloid or nutritional deficiencies.

The characteristic cataract in the Afghan hound begins as equatorial lens vacuoles in dogs from 4 months to 2 years of age. The opacities then extend into the anterior and posterior cortices. Rapid progression can occur with visual impairment in young adults. Test breedings have been done which support a hereditary basis; however, the exact mode of inheritance is unknown.

Other Conditions Under Consideration

C.   Marginal corneal degeneration

A white band-shaped vascularized opacity occurring in one or both eyes adjacent to the limbus. There is a clear area of cornea between the band and the limbus.

References

1.   ACVO Genetics Committee, 1992 and/or Data from CERF All-Breeds Report, 1991.

2.   Roberts SR, Helper LC: Cataracts in Afghan hounds. JAVMA 160: 427, 1972.

3.   Roberts SR: Hereditary cataracts. Vet Clin North Am 3: 433, 1973.

AIREDALE TERRIER

	DISORDER	INHERITANCE	REFERENCE	BREEDING ADVICE
A.	Distichiasis	Not defined	3	Breeder option
B.	Entropion	Not defined	2	Breeder option
C.	Corneal dystrophy	Not defined	1	NO
D.	Pannus	Not defined	3,4	Breeder option
E.	Progressive retinal atrophy	Not defined	5	NO

Description and Comments

A.   Distichiasis

Eyelashes abnormally located in the eyelid margin which may cause ocular irritation. Distichiasis may occur at any time in the life of a dog. It is difficult to make a strong recommendation with regard to breeding dogs with this entity. The hereditary basis has not been established although it seems probable due to the high incidence in some breeds. Reducing the incidence is a logical goal. When diagnosed, distichiasis should be recorded; breeding discretion is advised.

B.   Entropion

A conformational defect resulting in an "in-rolling" of one or more of the eyelids which may cause ocular irritation. It is likely that entropion is influenced by several genes (polygenic), defining the skin and other structures which make up the eyelids, the amount and weight of the skin covering the head and face, the orbital contents, and the conformation of the skull.

C.   Corneal dystrophy

A non-inflammatory corneal opacity (white to gray) present in one or more of the corneal layers; usually inherited and bilateral.

23

D.   Pannus / Chronic Superficial Keratitis

A bilateral disease of the cornea which usually starts as a grayish haze to the ventral or ventrolateral cornea, followed by the formation of a vascularized subepithelial growth that begins to spread toward the central cornea; pigmentation follows the vascularization. If severe, vision impairment occurs.

E.   Progressive Retinal Atrophy (PRA)

A degenerative disease of the retinal visual cells which progresses to blindness. This abnormality may be detected by electroretinogram before it is apparent clinically. In all breeds studied to date, PRA is recessively inherited.

Other Conditions Under Consideration

F.   Cataract

Lens opacity which may affect one or both eyes and may involve the lens partially or completely. In cases where cataracts are complete and affect both eyes, blindness results. The prudent approach is to assume cataracts to be hereditary except in cases known to be associated with trauma, other causes of ocular inflammation, specific metabolic diseases, persistent pupillary membranes, persistent hyaloid or nutritional deficiencies.

G.   Retinal Dysplasia

Abnormal development of the retina present at birth and recognized to have three forms:

1) Retinal dysplasia - **folds**: linear, triangular, curved or curvilinear foci of retinal folding that may be single or multiple.
2) Retinal dysplasia - **geographic**: any irregularly shaped area of abnormal retinal development, representing changes not accountable by simple folding.
3) Retinal dysplasia - **detachment**: either of the above described forms of retinal dysplasia associated with separation (detachment) of the retina.

The two latter forms are associated with vision impairment or blindness. Retinal dysplasia is known to be inherited in many breeds. The genetic relationship between the three forms of the disease is not known for all breeds.

Complete congenital detachment of the retina in the Airedale has been reported by Keller (5). All dogs had white hairs in the coat which may be a significant marker.

H.   Sclero-uveitis

An inflammatory disease of the sclera and uvea; the condition may be serious enough to cause blindness.

References

1.   Dice PF: Corneal dystrophy in the Airedale. Proc Am Coll Vet Ophthalmol, Fifth Annual Scientific Program, 1974: 80-86.

2.   Hodgman SFJ: Abnormalities and defects in pedigree dogs I. An investigation into the existence of abnormalities in pedigree dogs in the British Isles. J Small Anim Pract 4:447, 1963.

3.   ACVO Genetics Committee, 1992 and/or Data from CERF All-Breeds Report, 1991.

4.   Rubin LF: Inherited Eye Diseases in Purebred Dogs. Williams and Wilkins, Baltimore, 1989, pp.5-7.

5.   Priester WA: Canine progressive retinal atrophy. Occurrence by age, breed and sex. Am J Vet Res 35:571, 1974.

6.   Keller W, Blanchard G, Krehbiel J: Congenital dysplasia in a canine eye: a case report. J Am Anim Hosp Assoc 8:29, 1972.

AKITA

	DISORDER	INHERITANCE	REFERENCE	BREEDING ADVICE
A.	Uveitis/ Dermatologic syndrome	Not defined	1-4	Breeder option
B.	Multiple ocular defects	Not defined	5	NO
C.	Progressive Retinal Atrophy	Not defined	6,7	NO

Description and Comments

A.   Uveitis/Dermatologic Syndrome

The uveitis/dermatologic syndrome (Vogt-Koyanagi-Harada-like syndrome) is an immune-mediated disease in which melanocyte containing tissue (uvea and skin) is affected. Typical clinical presentation is bilateral anterior uveitis that may be associated with dermal depigmentation. Although the mode of inheritance has not been identified, there is a distinct breed predilection for the Akita.

B.   Multiple ocular defects

Multiple ocular defects consisting of microphthalmia, congenital cataracts, posterior lenticonus, and retinal dysplasia have been described in 3 litters of Akita puppies. Cataracts were nuclear and cortical in location. Retinal dysplasia was characterized by retinal folds and rosettes in the tapetal fundus. An autosomal recessive mode of inheritance is suspected but not proven.

C.   Progressive Retinal Atrophy (PRA)

A degenerative disease of the retinal visual cells which progresses to blindness. This abnormality may be detected by electroretinogram before it is apparent clinically. In all breeds studied to date, PRA is recessively inherited.

References

1. Kern TJ et al: Uveitis associated with poliosis and dermal depigmentation in dogs. J Am Vet Med Assoc 187:408, 1985.

2. Bussanich J: Granulomatous panuveitis and dermal depigmentation in dogs. J Am Anim Hosp Assoc 22:121, 1986.

3. Romatowski J: A uveodermatological syndrome in an Akita dog. J Am Anim Hosp Assoc 21:777, 1985.

4. Asakura I: Harada syndrome (uveitis diffusa acuta) in the dog. Japanese J Vet Med 673:445, 1977.

5. Laratta LJ et al: Multiple ocular defects in the Akita dog. Trans Fifteenth Ann Sci Prg Am Col Vet Ophthalmol, 1984, p158.

6. Otoole DO, Roberts S: Generalized progressive retinal atrophy in two Akita dogs. Vet Pathol 21:457, 1984.

7. Paulsen ME et al: Progressive retinal atrophy in a colony of Akita dogs. Trans Nineteenth Ann Sci Prog Am Col Vet Ophthal, 1988, p1.

ALASKAN MALAMUTE

	DISORDER	INHERITANCE	REFERENCE	BREEDING ADVICE
A.	Cataract	Not defined	1,3	NO
B.	Hemeralopia	Autosomal recessive	2	NO
C.	Progressive Retinal Atrophy	Not defined	1,3	NO
D.	Glaucoma	Not defined	1,3	NO

Descriptions and Comments

A. Cataract

Lens opacity which may affect one or both eyes and may involve the lens partially or completely. In cases where cataracts are complete and affect both eyes, blindness results. The prudent approach is to assume cataracts to be hereditary except in cases known to be associated with trauma, other causes of ocular inflammation, specific metabolic diseases, persistent pupillary membranes, persistent hyaloid or nutritional deficiencies.

B. Hemeralopia

A condition of day blindness. Dogs are blind in bright light but remain visual in dim/dark light.

C. Progressive Retinal Atrophy (PRA)

A degenerative disease of the retinal visual cells which progresses to blindness. This abnormality may be detected by electroretinogram before it is apparent clinically. In all breeds studied to date, PRA is recessively inherited.

D.   Glaucoma

An elevation of intraocular pressure (IOP) which, when sustained, causes intraocular damage resulting in blindness. The elevated IOP occurs because the fluid cannot leave through the iridocorneal angle. Diagnosis and classification of glaucoma require measurement of IOP (tonometry) and examination of the iridocorneal angle (gonioscopy). Neither of these tests are part of a routine breed eye screening exam.

References

1.   Rubin L: Inherited Eye Diseases in Purebred Dogs. Williams and Wilkins, 1989, p10.

2.   Rubin LF, Bourne TKR, Lord LH: Hemeralopia in dogs: heredity of hemeralopia in Alaska Malamutes. Am J Vet Res 28:355, 1967.

3.   ACVO Genetics Committee, 1992 and/or Data from CERF All-Breeds Report, 1991.

AMERICAN STAFFORDSHIRE TERRIER***

	DISORDER	INHERITANCE	REFERENCE	BREEDING ADVICE
A.	Entropion	Not defined	--	Breeder option
B.	Cataract	Not defined	1,2	NO
C.	Persistent Hyperplastic Primary Vitreous	Not defined	3	NO

*** Please note that since 1972 the AKC considers the Staffordshire Bull Terrier a <u>different</u> breed than the American Staffordshire Terrier. Since the latter breed evolved from the former, it is possible that the same genetic diseases exist in both. To date there are no specific reports of inherited eye diseases in the American Staffordshire Terrier.

Description and Comments

A.   Entropion

A conformational defect resulting in "in-rolling" of one or more of the eyelids which may cause ocular irritation. It is likely that entropion is influenced by several genes (polygenic), defining the skin and other structures which make up the eyelids, the amount and weight of the skin covering the head and face, the orbital contents and the conformation of the skull. Selection should be directed against entropion and toward a head conformation that minimizes or eliminates the likelihood of the defect.

B.   Cataract

Lens opacity which may affect one or both eyes and may involve the lens partially or completely. In cases where cataracts are complete and affect both eyes, blindness results. The prudent approach is to assume cataracts to be hereditary except in cases known to be associated with trauma, other causes of ocular inflammation, specific metabolic diseases, persistent pupillary membrane, persistent hyaloid or nutritional deficiencies.

In this breed, cataracts usually develop by one year of age. There is initial opacification of the suture lines progressing to nuclear and cortical cataract formation; complete cataracts and blindness develop by three years of age. A simple autosomal recessive mode of inheritance has been proposed; however, the genetics have not been defined and additional studies will be required.

C.   Persistent Hyperplastic Primary Vitreous (PHPV)

A congenital defect resulting from abnormalities in the development and regression of the hyaloid artery (the primary vitreous) and the interaction of this blood vessel with the posterior lens capsule/cortex during embryogenesis.

The majority of affected dogs have a retrolental fibrovascular plaque and variable lenticular defects which include posterior lenticonus/globus, colobomata, intralenticular hemorrhage and/or secondary cataracts. Vision impairment may result. The disease is an inherited disorder in the breed, but the mode of inheritance has not been defined. The results of current studies cannot rule out autosomal recessive or a dominant trait with incomplete penetrance.

References

1.   Barnett KC: Hereditary cataracts in the dog. J Small Anim Pract 19:109, 1978.

2.   Barnett KC: The diagnosis and differential diagnosis of cataracts in the dog. J Small Anim Pract 26:305, 1985.

3.   Leon A et al: Hereditary persistent hyperplastic primary vitreous in the Staffordshire Bull Terrier. JAAHA 22:765, 1986.

AMERICAN WATER SPANIEL

	DISORDER	INHERITANCE	REFERENCE	BREEDING ADVICE
A.	Cataract	Not defined	1	NO
B.	Retinal dysplasia - folds	Not defined	1	Breeder option

Description and Comments

A. Cataract

Lens opacity which may affect one or both eyes and may involve the lens partially or completely. In cases where cataracts are complete and affect both eyes, blindness results. The prudent approach is to assume cataracts to be hereditary except in cases known to be associated with trauma, other causes of ocular inflammation, specific metabolic diseases, persistent pupillary membrane, persistent hyaloid or nutritional deficiencies. Opacities of the anterior lens sutures have been reported in dogs less than 1 year of age.

B. Retinal Dysplasia

Abnormal development of the retina present at birth and recognized to have three forms:

1) Retinal dysplasia - **folds**: linear, triangular, curved or curvilinear foci of retinal folding that may be single or multiple.
2) Retinal dysplasia - **geographic**: any irregularly shaped area of abnormal retinal development, representing changes not accountable by simple folding.
3) Retinal dysplasia - **detachment**: either of the above described forms of retinal dysplasia associated with separation (detachment) of the retina.

The two latter forms are associated with vision impairment or blindness. Retinal dysplasia is known to be inherited in many breeds. The genetic relationship between the three forms of the disease is not known for all breeds.

References

There are no references providing detailed descriptions of hereditary ocular conditions of the American Water Spaniel breed. The conditions listed above are generally recognized to exist in this breed, as evidenced by repeated references made in general texts.

1.   ACVO Genetics Committee, 1992 and/or Data from CERF All-Breeds Report, 1991.

AUSTRALIAN CATTLE DOG
(Queensland Blue Heeler)

	DISORDER	INHERITANCE	REFERENCE	BREEDING ADVICE
A.	Progressive Retinal Atrophy	Not defined	--	NO
B.	Lens luxation	Not defined	--	NO
C.	Cataract	Not defined	1	NO

Description and Comments

A.   Progressive Retinal Atrophy (PRA)

A degenerative disease of the retinal visual cells which progresses to blindness. This abnormality may be detected by electroretinogram before it is apparent clinically. In all breeds studied to date, PRA is recessively inherited.

There are cases reported in the United States and Australia. Animals at the 3-5 year age range have had ophthalmoscopically typical signs of diffuse retinal degeneration which can be confirmed by electroretinography. Clinically there were only subtle signs of night blindness in the younger animals. Owners have reported obvious night and day blindness in animals at 5-6 years of age. Clinical experiences of Australian clinicians indicate the disease is a significant problem. There is no referenced proof of the mode of inheritance. However, it is presumed to be an autosomal recessive trait based on studies of similar disease in other breeds. Some ACVO diplomates have indicated that there may be more than one manifestation of the disease: an early emerging disease (2-4 years of age) and a later disease (5-6 year of age). Because of the significance of blindness, suspicious and affected animals are not to be recommended for breeding foundation. Parents of affected animals should be presumed to be carriers and siblings of affected animals should not be used as breed foundation.

B.   Luxated lens

Partial (subluxation) or complete displacement of the lens from the normal anatomic site behind the pupil. Lens luxation not associated with trauma or inflammation is presumed to be inherited. Lens luxation may result in elevated intraocular pressure (glaucoma) causing vision impairment or blindness.

Cases have been reported in Australia (J. Smith), but no references have been found. The lens luxates at middle age and is often found with concurrent glaucoma.

C.   Cataract

Lens opacity which may affect one or both eyes and may involve the lens partially or completely. In cases where cataracts are complete and affect both eyes, blindness results. The prudent approach is to assume cataracts to be hereditary except in cases known to be associated with trauma, other causes of ocular inflammation, specific metabolic diseases, persistent pupillary membrane, persistent hyaloid or nutritional deficiencies.

Other Conditions Under Consideration

D.   Retinal dysplasia

Abnormal development of the retina present at birth and recognized to have three forms:

1) Retinal dysplasia - **folds**: linear, triangular, curved or curvilinear foci of retinal folding that may be single or multiple.
2) Retinal dysplasia - **geographic**: any irregularly shaped area of abnormal retinal development, representing changes not accountable by simple folding.
3) Retinal dysplasia - **detachment**: either of the above described forms of retinal dysplasia associated with separation (detachment) of the retina.

The two latter forms are associated with vision impairment or blindness. Retinal dysplasia is known to be inherited in many breeds. The genetic relationship between the three forms of the disease is not known for all breeds.

E.   Persistent hyperplastic primary vitreous (PHPV)

A congenital defect resulting from abnormalities in the development and regression of the hyaloid artery (the primary vitreous) and the interaction of this blood vessel with the posterior lens capsule/cortex during embryogenesis.

This condition is often associated with **persistent tunica vasculosa lentis (PTVL)** which results from failure of regression of the embryologic vascular network which surrounds the developing lens.

F.   Vitreal degeneration

A liquefaction of the vitreous gel which may predispose to retinal detachment.

G.   Persistent pupillary membrane (PPM)

Persistent blood vessel remnants in the anterior chamber of the eye which fail to regress normally in the neonatal period. These strands may bridge from iris to iris, iris to cornea, iris to lens, or form sheets of tissue in the anterior chamber. The last three forms pose the greatest threat to vision and when severe, vision impairment or blindness may occur.

References

There are no references providing detailed descriptions of hereditary ocular conditions of the Australian Cattle Dog breed. The conditions listed above are generally recognized to exist in this breed, as evidenced by repeated references made in general texts.

1.   ACVO Genetics Committee, 1992 and/or Data from CERF All-Breeds Report, 1991.

AUSTRALIAN KELPIE

	DISORDER	INHERITANCE	REFERENCE	BREEDING ADVICE
A.	Progressive retinal atrophy	Not defined	1	NO

Description and Comments

A. Progressive Retinal Atrophy (PRA)

A degenerative disease of the retinal visual cells which progresses to blindness. This abnormality may be detected by electroretinogram before it is apparent clinically. In all breeds studied to date, PRA is recessively inherited.

References

There are no references providing detailed descriptions of hereditary ocular conditions of the Australian Kelpie breed. The conditions listed above are generally recognized to exist in this breed, as evidenced by repeated references made in general texts.

1. ACVO Genetics Committee, 1992 and/or Data from CERF All-Breeds Report, 1991.

AUSTRALIAN SHEPHERD

	DISORDER	INHERITANCE	REFERENCE	BREEDING ADVICE
A.	Microphthalmia/ multiple ocular defects	Not defined	1,2,3,4	NO
B.	Ocular coloboma/ staphyloma without microphthalmia	Not defined	4	NO
C.	Cataract	Not defined	5	NO
D.	Choroidal hypoplasia, +/- coloboma, +/- retinal detachment	Not defined	6	NO

Description and Comments

A.   Microphthalmia and associated ocular defects

Microphthalmia is a congenital defect characterized by a small eye with associated defects of the cornea, iris (coloboma), anterior chamber, lens (cataract) and/or retina (dysplasia). In the Australian Shepherd, this condition is usually associated with merling. The eyes of affected homozygous merle (usually white) dogs have extreme forms of this entity and are usually blind at birth. Affected heterozygous merle-coated dogs demonstrate less severe manifestations.

B.   Ocular coloboma/staphyloma unassociated with microphthalmia

A coloboma is a congenital defect which may affect the iris, choroid or optic disc. Iris colobomas are seen as notches in the pupillary margin. Scleral ectasia is defined as a congenital thinning and secondary distention of the sclera; when lined by uveal tissue it is called a staphyloma. These may be anteriorly located, apparent as a bulge beneath the upper eyelid or posteriorly located, requiring visualization with an ophthalmoscope. These conditions may or may not be genetically related to the same anomalies seen associated with microphthalmia (entity "A" above).

C.   Cataract

Lens opacity which may affect one or both eyes and may involve the lens partially or completely. In cases where cataracts are complete and affect both eyes, blindness results. The prudent approach is to assume cataracts to be hereditary except in cases known to be associated with trauma, other causes of ocular inflammation, specific metabolic diseases, persistent pupillary membrane, persistent hyaloid or nutritional deficiencies.

C.   Choroidal hypoplasia

A congenital defect in which the choroid develops incompletely. The clinical appearance is similar to the same condition reported in Collies and Shetland Sheepdogs.

References

1.   Gelatt KN, McGill LD: Clinical characteristics of microphthalmia with colobomas of the Australian shepherd dog. J Am Vet Med Assoc 162:393, 1971.

2.   Gelatt KN, Veith LA: Hereditary multiple ocular anomalies in Australian shepherd dogs. Vet Med Small Anim Clin 654:9, 1970.

3.   Cook CS, Burling K, Nelson EJ: Embryogenesis of posterior segment colobomas in the Australian shepherd dog. Prog in Vet Comp Ophthalmol 1: 163, 1991.

4.   Bertram T, Coiqnoul F, Cheville N: Ocular dysgenesis in Australian shepherd dogs. J Am Anim Hosp Assoc 20:177, 1984.

5.   ACVO Genetics Committee, 1992 and/or Data from CERF All-Breeds Report, 1991.

6.   Rubin LF, Nelson EJ, Sharp CA: Collie eye anomaly in Australian shepherd dogs. Prog in Vet Comp Ophthalmol 1: 105, 1991.

BASENJI

	DISORDER	INHERITANCE	REFERENCE	BREEDING ADVICE
A.	Persistent pupillary membranes	Not defined	1,2,3	NO
B.	Progressive Retinal Atrophy	Not defined	4,5	NO
C.	Optic nerve coloboma	Not defined	1	NO

Description and Comments

A. Persistent pupillary membranes (PPM)

Persistent blood vessel remnants in the anterior chamber of the eye which fail to regress normally in the neonatal period. These strands may bridge from iris to iris, iris to cornea, iris to lens, or form sheets of tissue in the anterior chamber. The last three forms pose the greatest threat to vision and when severe, vision impairment or blindness may occur.

B. Progressive Retinal Atrophy

A degenerative disease of the retinal visual cells which progresses to blindness. This abnormality may be detected by electroretinogram before it is apparent clinically. In all breeds studied to date, PRA is recessively inherited.

C. Optic nerve coloboma

A congenital cavity in the optic nerve which, if large, may cause blindness or vision impairment.

Other Conditions Under Consideration

D.   Cataract

Lens opacity which may affect one or both eyes and may involve the lens partially or completely. In cases where cataracts are complete and affect both eyes, blindness results. The prudent approach is to assume cataracts to be hereditary except in cases known to be associated with trauma, other causes of ocular inflammation, specific metabolic diseases, persistent pupillary membrane, persistent hyaloid or nutritional deficiencies.

References

1.   Barnett KC, Knight GC: Persistent pupillary membrane and associated defects in the Basenji. Vet Rec 85:242, 1969.

2.   Mason TA: Persistent pupillary membranes in the Basenji. Austral Vet J 52:343, 1976.

3.   Roberts SR, Bistner SI: Persistent pupillary membrane in Basenji dogs. J Am Vet Med Assoc 153:571, 1968.

4.   Priester WA: Canine progressive retinal atrophy. Occurrence by age, breed and sex. Am J Vet Res 35:571, 1974.

5.   ACVO Genetics Committee, 1992 and/or Data from CERF All-Breeds Report, 1991.

BASSET HOUND

	DISORDER	INHERITANCE	REFERENCE	BREEDING ADVICE
A.	Glaucoma	Not defined	1,2	NO
B.	Ectropion	Not defined	--	Breeder option
C.	Entropion	Not defined	--	Breeder option

Description and Comments

A.   Glaucoma

Glaucoma is characterized by an elevation of intraocular pressure which, when sustained, causes intraocular damage resulting in blindness. The elevated intraocular pressure occurs because the fluid cannot leave through the iridocorneal angle. Diagnosis and classification of glaucoma requires measurement of IOP (tonometry) and examination of the iridocorneal angle (gonioscopy). Neither of these tests are part of a routine breed eye screening exam.

Some Basset Hounds have an abnormality of the iridocorneal angle termed goniodysgenesis. This abnormality is not visible during routine ophthalmologic examination using an indirect ophthalmoscope or a slitlamp microscope. There appears to be an association between goniodysgenesis and glaucoma, but the mechanism by which the angle defect results in glaucoma has not been determined. It is suspected that mild to severe anterior uveitis impairs outflow of aqueous through the small perforations that are present in the sheet of tissue in the iridocorneal angle; this results in a secondary and often irreversible rise in intraocular pressure that causes blindness. The inheritance of goniodysgenesis in the Basset Hound is not known. Until the inheritance is determined, control should be aimed at removing from breeding dogs that have glaucoma and have goniodysgenesis, as well as those dogs that produce progeny affected with glaucoma.

B.   Ectropion

A conformational defect resulting in eversion of the eyelids, which may cause ocular irritation. It is likely that ectropion is influenced by several genes (polygenic) defining the skin and other structures which make up the eyelids, the amount and weight of the skin covering the head and face, the orbital contents and the conformation of the skull.

In the Basset Hound, ectropion is associated with an exceptionally large palpebral fissure (macroblepharon) and laxity of the canthal structures.   Central lower lid ectropion is often associated with entropion of the adjacent lid segment. This causes severe ocular irritation.

It is acknowledged that factors other than genetics may play a role or be the cause of entropion and/or ectropion. However, when non-genetic factors can be ruled out, selection should be directed to a more normal head conformation that minimizes or eliminates the likelihood of the defects.

C.   Entropion

A conformational defect resulting in an "in-rolling" of one or more of the eyelids which may cause ocular irritation. It is likely that entropion is influenced by several genes (polygenic) defining the skin and other structures which make up the eyelids, the amount and weight of the skin covering the head and face, the orbital contents and the conformation of the skull.

References

1.   Martin CL and Wyman M: Glaucoma in the Basset Hound. J Am Vet Med Assoc 155:1320, 1968.

2.   Wyman M and Ketring K: Congenital glaucoma in the Basset hound: a biologic model. Trans Am Acad Ophth and Otol 81: OP-645, 1976.

BEAGLE

	DISORDER	INHERITANCE	REFERENCE	BREEDING ADVICE
A.	Microphthalmia and multiple congenital ocular anomalies	See below	1,2,3	NO
B.	Glaucoma	Autosomal recessive	4,5	NO
C.	Prolapse of gland of third eyelid	Not defined	--	Breeder option
D.	Cataract	Not defined	1	NO
E.	Tapetal degeneration	Autosomal recessive	6	Breeder option
F.	Progressive retinal atrophy	Not defined	--	NO

Description and Comments

A.   Microphthalmia and multiple congenital ocular anomalies

A developmental anomaly in which the eyeball is abnormally small. This is often associated with other ocular malformations, including defects of the cornea, anterior chamber, lens, and/or retina.

In the Beagle, the condition may be present unilaterally or bilaterally and is characterized by a small globe and associated ocular defects which are variable. Several forms of the condition, all apparently different, are recognized:

44

1) In one study, complete lens opacities were noted by 5-6 months of age; the severity of the cataract correlated closely with the extent of microphthalmia. Severely microphthalmic eyes also had multiple retinal folds. The disorder appeared to be inherited; the exact mode was not fully defined, although an X-linked disorder could be ruled out.

2) A different form of microphthalmia is recognized in association with microphakia and persistent pupillary membrane (PPM). Based on a limited pedigree of one cross, a dominant inheritance was proposed; heterozygotes have PPM and microphakia / cataract and homozygous affected show microphthalmia and multiple congenital ocular anomalies.

3) A third form of microphthalmia is recognized in the breed. This condition is usually unilateral and the fellow eye is normal. The mode of inheritance has not been defined, but autosomal recessive inheritance is suspected.

B.   Glaucoma

Glaucoma is an elevation of intraocular pressure (IOP) which, when sustained, causes intraocular damage resulting in blindness. The elevated IOP occurs because the fluid cannot leave through the iridocorneal angle. Diagnosis and classification of glaucoma requires measurement of IOP (tonometry) and examination of the iridocorneal angle (gonioscopy). Neither of these tests are part of a routine breed eye screening exam.

Primary open angle glaucoma is present in the breed, and extensive breeding studies have demonstrated its inheritance as autosomal recessive. By one year of age, the intraocular pressure (IOP) is elevated, but the filtration angle is open (early glaucoma). Animals with moderate glaucoma show sustained elevations of IOP, focal disinsertions of the lens zonules and focal closures of the iridocorneal angle. Later the globe enlarges, the lens luxates and the eyes become blind and show the effects of chronic glaucoma.

C.   Prolapse of the gland of the third eyelid

Protrusion of the tear gland associated with the third eyelid. The mode of inheritance of this disorder is unknown. The exposed gland may become irritated. Commonly referred to as "cherry eye". In the Beagle, there seems to be an association between this condition and keratoconjunctivitis sicca (KCS).

D. Cataracts

Lens opacity which may affect one or both eyes and may involve the lens partially or completely. In cases where cataracts are complete and affect both eyes, blindness results. The prudent approach is to assume cataracts to be hereditary except in cases known to be associated with trauma, other causes of ocular inflammation, specific metabolic diseases, persistent pupillary membrane, persistent hyaloid or nutritional deficiencies.

Several different types of cataract (anterior capsular, posterior cortical, other) have been reported in the breed, but the inheritance of the defects, if they are inherited, is unknown (see reference #1 for review). When one considers that this breed, particularly the laboratory-bred beagle, has been the subject of extensive ophthalmological examination, the low incidence of cataracts is surprising.

E. Tapetal degeneration

The tapetum lucidum is a modified choroidal structure present in the eyes of many animals that have good night vision. In Beagles there is a recessively inherited defect of the tapetal layer. Absence of this layer is determined by ophthalmoscopy which shows that the fundus has a uniform reddish coloration. The degeneration of the tapetum occurs as a result of abnormal postnatal development of this structure. The degeneration of the tapetum does not affect vision and does not result in functional or structural damage to the retina. As such, the condition probably represents an insignificant inherited variation of no functional significance.

F. Progressive Retinal Atrophy (PRA)

A degenerative disease of the retinal visual cells which progresses to blindness. This abnormality may be detected by electroretinogram before it is apparent clinically. In all breeds studied to date, PRA is recessively inherited. The disease in the Beagle has not been characterized sufficiently to establish the disease frequency, the disease mechanism, or the age when early diagnosis by ophthalmoscopy and/or electroretinography is possible.

References

1. Rubin L: Inherited Eye Diseases in Purebred Dogs. Williams and Wilkins, Baltimore, 1989, pp 22-30.

2. Andersen AC, Shultz FT: Inherited (congenital) cataract in the dog. Am J Path 34: 965, 1958.

3.   American Kennel Club Genetic Disease Registry. Univ of Penn, 1989.

4.   Gelatt KN, Gum GG: Inheritance of glaucoma in the beagle. Am J Vet Res 42: 1691, 1981.

5.   Gelatt KN et al: Clinical manifestations of inherited glaucoma in the beagle. Invest Ophthalmol Vis Sci 16: 1135, 1977.

6.   Burns MS et al: Development of hereditary tapetal degeneration in the beagle dog. Curr Eye Res 7:103, 1988.

BEARDED COLLIE

	DISORDER	INHERITANCE	REFERENCE	BREEDING ADVICE
A.	Cataract	Not defined	1	NO
B.	Retinal dysplasia - folds	Not defined	2	Breeder option

Description and Comments

A.   Cataract

Lens opacity which may affect one or both eyes and may involve the lens partially or completely. In cases where cataracts are complete and affect both eyes, blindness results. The prudent approach is to assume cataracts to be hereditary except in cases known to be associated with trauma, other causes of ocular inflammation, specific metabolic diseases, persistent pupillary membrane, persistent hyaloid or nutritional deficiencies.

B.   Retinal dysplasia

Abnormal development of the retina present at birth and recognized to have three forms:

1) Retinal dysplasia - **folds**: linear, triangular, curved or curvilinear foci of retinal folding that may be single or multiple.
2) Retinal dysplasia - **geographic**: any irregularly shaped area of abnormal retinal development representing changes not accountable by simple folding.
3) Retinal dysplasia - **detachment**: either of the above described forms of retinal dysplasia associated with separation (detachment) of the retina.

The two latter forms are associated with vision impairment or blindness. Retinal dysplasia is known to be inherited in many breeds. The genetic relationship between the three forms of the disease is not known for all breeds.

References

1. ACVO Genetics Committee, 1992 and/or Data from CERF All-Breeds Report, 1991.

2. Bedford PGC: Multifocal retinal dysplasia in the rottweiler. Vet Rec 111: 304, 1982.

BEDLINGTON TERRIER

	DISORDER	INHERITANCE	REFERENCE	BREEDING ADVICE
A.	Microphthalmia	Not defined	1	NO
B.	Distichiasis	Not defined	1	Breeder option
C.	Imperforate lacrimal punctum	Not defined	2	Breeder option
D.	Cataract	Not defined	1	NO
E.	Retinal dysplasia - folds	Not defined	1	Breeder option
F.	Retinal dysplasia - geographic - detachment	Autosomal recessive	3	NO

Description and Comments

A.   Microphthalmia

Microphthalmia is a congenital defect characterized by a small eye with associated defects of the cornea, iris (coloboma), anterior chamber, lens (cataract) and/or retina.

B.   Distichiasis

Eyelashes abnormally located in the eyelid margin which may cause ocular irritation. Distichiasis may occur at any time in the life of a dog. It is difficult to make a strong recommendation with regard to breeding dogs with this entity. The hereditary basis has not been established although it seems probable due to the high incidence in some breeds. Reducing the incidence is a logical goal. When diagnosed, distichiasis should be recorded. Breeding discretion is advised.

C.   Imperforate lacrimal punctum

A congenital condition in which the opening of the nasolacrimal drainage system fails to develop resulting in epiphora or spillover of tears onto the face.

D.   Cataract

Lens opacity which may affect one or both eyes and may involve the lens partially or completely. In cases where cataracts are complete and affect both eyes, blindness results. The prudent approach is to assume cataracts to be hereditary except in cases known to be associated with trauma, other causes of ocular inflammation, specific metabolic diseases, persistent pupillary membranes, persistent hyaloid or nutritional deficiencies.

E,F.   Retinal dysplasia

Abnormal development of the retina present at birth and recognized to have three forms:

    1) Retinal dysplasia - **folds**: linear, triangular, curved or curvilinear foci of retinal folding that may be single or multiple.
    2) Retinal dysplasia - **geographic**: any irregularly shaped area of abnormal retinal development representing changes not accountable by simple folding.
    3) Retinal dysplasia - **detachment**: either of the above described forms of retinal dysplasia associated with separation (detachment) of the retina.

The two latter forms are associated with vision impairment or blindness. Retinal dysplasia is known to be inherited in many breeds. The genetic relationship between the three forms of the disease is not known for all breeds.

Other Conditions Under Consideration

G.   Lens Luxation

Partial (subluxation) or complete displacement of the lens from the normal anatomic site behind the pupil. Lens luxation not associated with trauma or inflammation is presumed to be inherited. Lens luxation may result in elevated intraocular pressure (glaucoma) causing vision impairment or blindness.

There is insufficient information regarding this disease entity in the Bedlington terrier to make a definitive recommendation.

References

1. ACVO Genetics Committee, 1992 and/or Data from CERF All-Breeds Report, 1991.

2. Gelatt KN: Pediatric ophthalmology in small animal practice. In Aguirre G (ed): The Veterinary Clinics of North America, Vol 3, No 3, WB Saunders Co, Philadelphia, 1973.

3. Rubin LF: Heredity of retinal dysplasia in the Bedlington terrier. J Am Vet Med Assoc 152:260, 1968.

BELGIAN MALINOIS

	DISORDER	INHERITANCE	REFERENCE	BREEDING ADVICE
A.	Progressive Retinal Atrophy	Not defined	1	NO

Description and Comments

A.   Progressive Retinal Atrophy (PRA)

A degenerative disease of the retinal visual cells which progresses to blindness. This abnormality may be detected by electroretinogram before it is apparent clinically. In all breeds studied to date, PRA is recessively inherited.

References

There are no references providing detailed descriptions of hereditary ocular conditions of the Belgian Malinois breed. The conditions listed above are generally recognized to exist in this breed, as evidenced by repeated references made in general texts.

1.   ACVO Genetics Committee, 1992 and/or Data from CERF All-Breeds Report, 1991.

BELGIAN SHEEPDOG

	DISORDER	INHERITANCE	REFERENCE	BREEDING ADVICE
A.	Retinopathy	Autosomal recessive	1	NO
B.	Pannus	Not defined	2	NO
C.	Cataract	Not defined	2	NO

Description and Comments

A. Retinopathy

A visual deficit seen as early as eight weeks of age. Vision is disturbed both in bright and dim light. Ophthalmoscopically multifocal areas of retinal thickening are seen. The disease seems to affect the retinal pigment epithelial and photoreceptor regions histologically.

B. Pannus

A bilateral disease of the cornea which usually starts as a grayish haze to the ventral or ventrolateral cornea, followed by the formation of a vascularized subepithelial growth that begins to spread toward the central cornea; pigmentation follows the vascularization. If severe, vision impairment occurs.

C. Cataract

Lens opacity which may affect one or both eyes and may involve the lens partially or completely. In cases where cataracts are complete and affect both eyes, blindness results. The prudent approach is to assume cataracts to be hereditary except in cases known to be associated with trauma, other causes of ocular inflammation, specific metabolic diseases, persistent pupillary membranes, persistent hyaloid or nutritional deficiencies.

The cataract seems to be triangular in the posterior polar region.

Other Conditions Under Consideration

D.   Progressive Retinal Atrophy (PRA)

A degenerative disease of the retinal visual cells which progresses to blindness. This abnormality may be detected by electroretinogram before it is apparent clinically. In all breeds studied to date, PRA is recessively inherited.

E.   Micropapilla

A small optic disc which is not associated with vision impairment. May be unable to differentiate from optic nerve hypoplasia on a routine (dilated) screening ophthalmoscopic exam.

References

1.   Wolf ED, Samuelson D: Retinopathy is a family of Belgium shepherds. Transactions of the Twelfth Annual Scientific Program of the American College of Veterinary Ophthalmologists, 1981, supplement.

2.   ACVO Genetics Committee, 1992 and/or Data from CERF All-Breeds Report, 1991.

BELGIAN TERVUREN

	DISORDER	INHERITANCE	REFERENCE	BREEDING ADVICE
A.	Cataract	Not defined	1	NO
B.	Micropapilla	Not defined	1	Breeder option
C.	Progressive Retinal Atrophy	Not defined	--	NO
D.	Pannus	Not defined	1	NO

Description and Comments

A.   Cataract

Lens opacity which may affect one or both eyes and may involve the lens partially or completely. In cases where cataracts are complete and affect both eyes, blindness results. The prudent approach is to assume cataracts to be hereditary except in cases known to be associated with trauma, other causes of ocular inflammation, specific metabolic diseases, persistent pupillary membranes, persistent hyaloid or nutritional deficiencies.

B.   Micropapilla

A small optic disc which is not associated with vision impairment. May be unable to differentiate from optic nerve hypoplasia on a routine (dilated) screening ophthalmoscopic exam.

C.   Progressive Retinal Atrophy (PRA)

A degenerative disease of the retinal visual cells which progresses to blindness. This abnormality may be detected by electroretinogram before it is apparent clinically. In all breeds studied to date, PRA is recessively inherited.

D. Pannus

A bilateral disease of the cornea which usually starts as a grayish haze to the ventral or ventrolateral cornea, followed by the formation of a vascularized subepithelial growth that begins to spread toward the central cornea; pigmentation follows the vascularization. If severe, vision impairment occurs.

Other Conditions Under Consideration

E. Optic nerve hypoplasia

A congenital defect of the optic nerve which causes blindness and abnormal pupil response in the affected eye. May be unable to differentiate from micropapilla on a routine (dilated) screening ophthalmoscopic exam.

References

There are no references providing detailed descriptions of hereditary ocular conditions of the Belgian Tervuren breed. The conditions listed above are generally recognized to exist in this breed, as evidenced by repeated references made in general texts.

1. ACVO Genetics Committee, 1992 and/or Data from CERF All-Breeds Report, 1991.

BERNESE MOUNTAIN DOG

	DISORDER	INHERITANCE	REFERENCE	BREEDING ADVICE
A.	Progressive Retinal Atrophy	Not defined	1	NO
B.	Cataract	Not defined	1	NO
C.	Entropion	Not defined	1	Breeder option

Description and Comments

A.   Progressive Retinal Atrophy (PRA)

A degenerative disease of the retinal visual cells which progresses to blindness. This abnormality may be detected by electroretinogram before it is apparent clinically. In all breeds studied to date, PRA is recessively inherited.

B.   Cataract

Lens opacity which may affect one or both eyes and may involve the lens partially or completely. In cases where cataracts are complete and affect both eyes, blindness results. The prudent approach is to assume cataracts to be hereditary except in cases known to be associated with trauma, other causes of ocular inflammation, specific metabolic diseases, persistent pupillary membranes, persistent hyaloid or nutritional deficiencies.

C.   Entropion

A conformational defect resulting in an "in-rolling" of one or more of the eyelids which may cause ocular irritation. It is likely that entropion is influenced by several genes (polygenic) defining the skin and other structures which make up the eyelids, the amount and weight of the skin covering the head and face, the orbital contents and the conformation of the skull.

References

There are no references providing detailed descriptions of hereditary ocular conditions of the Bernese Mountain Dog breed. The conditions listed above are generally recognized to exist in this breed, as evidenced by repeated references made in general texts.

1. ACVO Genetics Committee, 1992 and/or Data from CERF All-Breeds Report, 1991.

BICHON FRISE

	DISORDER	INHERITANCE	REFERENCE	BREEDING ADVICE
A.	Entropion	Not defined	--	Breeder option
B.	Corneal dystrophy	Not defined	--	Breeder option
C.	Cataract	Not defined	1	NO

Description and Comments

A.   Entropion

A conformational defect resulting in an "in-rolling" of one or more of the eyelids which may cause ocular irritation. It is likely that entropion is influenced by several genes (polygenic) defining the skin and other structures which make up the eyelids, the amount and weight of the skin covering the head and face, the orbital contents and the conformation of the skull.

B.   Corneal dystrophy

A non-inflammatory corneal opacity (white to gray) present in one or more of the corneal layers; usually inherited and bilateral.

C.   Cataract

Lens opacity which may affect one or both eyes and may involve the lens partially or completely. In cases where cataracts are complete and affect both eyes, blindness results. The prudent approach is to assume cataracts to be hereditary except in cases known to be associated with trauma, other causes of ocular inflammation, specific metabolic diseases, persistent pupillary membranes, persistent hyaloid or nutritional deficiencies.

References

There are no references providing detailed descriptions of hereditary ocular conditions of the Bichon Frise breed. The conditions listed above are generally recognized to exist in this breed, as evidenced by repeated references made in general texts.

1. ACVO Genetics Committee, 1992 and/or Data from CERF All-Breeds Report, 1991.

BLOODHOUND

	DISORDER	INHERITANCE	REFERENCE	BREEDING ADVICE
A.	Ectropion with macroblepharon	Not defined	1	Breeder option
B.	Entropion	Not defined	1	NO
C.	Prolapse of the gland of third eyelid	Not defined	2	Breeder option

Description and Comment

A.   Ectropion/macroblepharon

A conformational defect resulting in eversion of the eyelid(s), which may cause ocular irritation due to exposure. It is likely that ectropion is influenced by several genes (polygenic) defining the skin and other structures which make up the eyelids, the amount and weight of the skin covering the head and face, the orbital contents and the conformation of the skull.

In the Bloodhound, ectropion is associated with an exceptionally large palpebral fissure (ie, macroblepharon) and laxity of the canthal structures. Central lower lid ectropion is often associated with entropion of the adjacent lid. This causes severe ocular irritation.

B.   Entropion

A conformational defect resulting in an "in-rolling" of one or more of the eyelids which may cause ocular irritation. It is likely that entropion is influenced by several genes (polygenic) defining the skin and other structures which make up the eyelids, the amount and weight of the skin covering the head and face, the orbital contents and the conformation of the skull.

C.   Prolapse of the gland of the third eyelid

Protrusion of the tear gland associated with the third eyelid. The mode of inheritance of this disorder is unknown. The exposed gland may become irritated. Commonly referred to as "cherry eye".

References

1.   Barnett KC: Comparative aspects of canine hereditary eye disease. Adv Vet Sci Comp Med 20:39, 1976.

2.   ACVO Genetics Committee, 1992 and/or Data from CERF All-Breeds Report, 1991.

BORDER COLLIE

	DISORDER	INHERITANCE	REFERENCE	BREEDING ADVICE
A.	Lens luxation	Not defined	1	NO
B.	Central Progressive Retinal Atrophy	Not defined	2	NO
C.	Progressive Retinal Atrophy	Not defined	3	NO
D.	Collie Eye Anomaly	Not defined	4	NO

Description and Comments

A. Lens luxation

Partial (subluxation) or complete displacement of the lens from the normal anatomic site behind the pupil. Lens luxation not associated with trauma or inflammation is presumed to be inherited. Lens luxation may result in elevated intraocular pressure (glaucoma), causing vision impairment or blindness.

B. Central Progressive Retinal Atrophy (CPRA)

A progressive retinal degeneration in which photoreceptor degeneration occurs secondary to disease of the underlying pigment epithelium. Progression is slow and some animals may never lose vision. CPRA is a frequent occurrence in England, but is uncommon elsewhere.

C. Progressive Retinal Atrophy (PRA)

A degenerative disease of the retinal visual cells which progresses to blindness. This abnormality may be detected by electroretinogram before it is apparent clinically. In all breeds studied to date, PRA is recessively inherited.

D.   Collie Eye Anomaly (CEA)

A congenital syndrome of ocular anomalies seen in the collie and which includes choroidal hypoplasia, staphyloma, coloboma.

Other Conditions Under Consideration

E.   Distichiasis

Eyelashes abnormally located in the eyelid margin which may cause ocular irritation. Distichiasis may occur at any time in the life of a dog. It is difficult to make a strong recommendation with regard to breeding dogs with this entity. The hereditary basis has not been established, although it seems probable due to the high incidence in some breeds. Reducing the incidence is a logical goal. When diagnosed, distichiasis should be recorded; breeding discretion is advised.

F.   Corneal dystrophy

A non-inflammatory corneal opacity (white to gray) present in one or more of the corneal layers; usually inherited and bilateral.

G.   Cataract

Lens opacity which may affect one or both eyes and may involve the lens partially or completely. In cases where cataracts are complete and affect both eyes, blindness results. The prudent approach is to assume cataracts to be hereditary except in cases known to be associated with trauma, other causes of ocular inflammation, specific metabolic diseases, persistent pupillary membrane, persistent hyaloid or nutritional deficiencies.

References

1.   Foster SJ et al: Primary lens luxation in the Border collie. J Small Anim Pract 27:1, 1986.

2.   Barnett KC et al: The International Sheep Dog Society and progressive retinal atrophy. J Small Anim Pract 10:301, 1969.

3.   Barnett KC: Canine retinopathies II. The other breeds. J Small Anim Pract 6:185, 1965.

4.   Bedford PGC: Collie eye anomaly in the Border collie. Vet Rec 111:34, 1982.

BORDER TERRIER

	DISORDER	INHERITANCE	REFERENCE	BREEDING ADVICE
A.	Cataract	Not defined	1	NO
C.	Progressive Retinal Atrophy	Not defined	1	NO

Description and Comments

A.   Cataract

Lens opacity which may affect one or both eyes and may involve the lens partially or completely. In cases where cataracts are complete and affect both eyes, blindness results. The prudent approach is to assume cataracts to be hereditary except in cases known to be associated with trauma, other causes of ocular inflammation, specific metabolic diseases, persistent pupillary membranes, persistent hyaloid or nutritional deficiencies.

Cataracts in the Border Terrier have an onset of 3-5 years, are slowly progressive and are located in the posterior subcapsular region, starting along the suture lines. Vision impairment is uncommon.

C.   Progressive Retinal Atrophy (PRA)

A degenerative disease of the retinal visual cells which progresses to blindness. This abnormality may be detected by electroretinogram before it is apparent clinically. In all breeds studied to date, PRA is recessively inherited.

In the Border Terrier, PRA appears to be a rare condition in middle-aged dogs.

References

There are no references providing detailed descriptions of hereditary ocular conditions of the Border Terrier breed. The conditions listed above are generally recognized to exist in this breed, as evidenced by repeated references made in general texts.

1.   ACVO Genetics Committee, 1992 and/or Data from CERF All-Breeds Report, 1991.

BORZOI

	DISORDER	INHERITANCE	REFERENCE	BREEDING ADVICE
A.	Microphthalmia and congenital ocular anomalies	Not defined	1	NO
B.	Cataract	Not defined	--	NO
C.	Progressive Retinal Atrophy	Not defined	--	NO
D.	Retinal degeneration	Not defined	2	NO

Description and Comments

A. Microphthalmia and multiple congenital ocular anomalies

A congenital defect characterized by a small eye with associated defects of the cornea, anterior chamber, lens and/or retina. In several interrelated Borzois, microphthalmia has been reported often in association with multiple ocular anomalies. These include cataract, multifocal retinal dysplasia, and persistent pupillary membrane. The significance of the disorder to the breed or the mode of inheritance are unknown at this time. Similar congenital ocular defects that are likely to be inherited have been reported in other dog breeds.

B. Cataract

Lens opacity which may affect one or both eyes and may involve the lens partially or completely. In cases where cataracts are complete and affect both eyes, blindness results. The prudent approach is to assume cataracts to be hereditary except in cases known to be associated with trauma, other causes of ocular inflammation, specific metabolic diseases, persistent pupillary membranes, persistent hyaloid or nutritional deficiencies. The frequency and significance of cataracts in the breed is not known.

C.   Progressive Retinal Atrophy (PRA)

A degenerative disease of the retinal visual cells which progresses to blindness. This abnormality may be detected by electroretinogram before it is apparent clinically. In all breeds studied to date, PRA is recessively inherited.   The frequency and significance of PRA in the breed is unknown.   PRA in the Borzoi must be differentiated from Retinal Degeneration (see below).

D.   Retinal Degeneration

A unilateral or bilateral retinal disease that affects young and adult Borzois and which can be progressive. When bilateral, the ophthalmoscopic lesions are often asymmetrical, particularly in the early stages of the disease. Fundus examination shows initially single or multiple focal retinal lesions that appear active (inflammatory: locally infiltrative or granulomatous) or inactive. The lesions can progress resulting in widespread retinal atrophy. The end-stage ophthalmoscopic lesions vary and may appear indistinguishable from PRA, or may be more characteristic of an inflammatory retinopathy.   The asymmetry of the fundus abnormalities and the presence of retinochoroidal inflammatory lesions help to differentiate this disorder from PRA. The mode of inheritance of this disease is not known; however, studies of different families suggest that it is possibly inherited. An intriguing aspect of the disease has been the preponderance of affected males compared to females. This has been confirmed in a recent unpublished survey.

References

1.   Rubin LF: Inherited Eye Diseases in Purebred Dogs. Williams & Wilkins, Baltimore, 1989, p44.

2.   Scagliotti R and MacMillan A: Retinal degeneration in the Borzoi. A preliminary report. Trans Am Coll Vet Ophthal, 1977, p67.

3.   Laratta LJ, Riis RC, Kern TJ et al: Multiple congenital ocular defects in the Akita dog. Cornell Vet 75:381, 1985.

4.   Narfstrom K, Dubielzig R: Posterior lenticonus, cataracts and microphthalmia: Congenital ocular defects in the Cavalier King Charles spaniel. J Small Anim Pract 25:669, 1984.

5.   Lewis DG, Kelly DF and Sansom J: Congenital microphthalmia and other developmental ocular anomalies in the Doberman. J Small Anim Pract 27:559, 1986.

6.   Acland GM: Unpublished information, 1988/89.

BOSTON TERRIER

	DISORDER	INHERITANCE	REFERENCE	BREEDING ADVICE
A.	Endothelial dystrophy	Not defined	1,2	NO
B.	Cataract	Not defined	2,3	NO

Description and Comments

A. Corneal endothelial dystrophy

Corneal endothelial dystrophy is an abnormal loss of the inner lining of the cornea that causes progressive fluid retention (edema). With time the edema results in keratitis and decreased vision. This usually does not occur until the animal is older.

B. Cataract

Lens opacity which may affect one or both eyes and may involve the lens partially or completely. In cases where cataracts are complete and affect both eyes, blindness results. The prudent approach is to assume cataracts to be hereditary except in cases known to be associated with trauma, other causes of ocular inflammation, specific metabolic diseases, persistent pupillary membranes, persistent hyaloid or nutritional deficiencies.

Other Conditions Under Consideration

C. Iris cysts

Pigmented cysts arise from posterior pigmented epithelial cells of the iris and remain attached or break free, floating as pigmented spheres of various sizes and pigments in the anterior chamber. Some cysts tend to adhere to the posterior surface of the cornea. Rarely, cysts may be numerous enough to impair vision. The mode of inheritance is unknown.

D.   Vitreal degeneration and/or prolapse

Vitreous degeneration is a liquefaction of the vitreous gel which may predispose to retinal detachment. Vitreous prolapse may occur when the liquefied vitreous prolapses into the anterior chamber. This may predispose the animal to glaucoma by blockage of the filtration angle or by pupillary blockade.

References

1.   Martin CL, Dice PF: Corneal endothelial dystrophy in the dog. J Am Anim Hosp Assoc 18:327, 1982.

2.   Rubin L: Inherited Eye Diseases in Purebred Dogs. Williams & Wilkins, 1989.

3.   Curtis R: Late onset cataract in the Boston terrier. Vet Res 115:755, 1984.

BOUVIER DES FLANDRES

	DISORDER	INHERITANCE	REFERENCE	BREEDING ADVICE
A.	Cataracts	Not defined	1	NO
B.	Entropion	Not defined	2	Breeder option
C.	Glaucoma	Not defined	3,4	NO

Description and Comments

A.   Cataracts

Lens opacity which may affect one or both eyes and may involve the lens partially or completely. In cases where cataracts are complete and affect both eyes, blindness results. The prudent approach is to assume cataracts to be hereditary except in cases known to be associated with trauma, other causes of ocular inflammation, specific metabolic diseases, persistent pupillary membranes, persistent hyaloid or nutritional deficiencies.

B.   Entropion

A conformational defect resulting in an "in-rolling" of one or more of the eyelids which may cause ocular irritation. It is likely that entropion is influenced by several genes (polygenic) defining the skin and other structures which make up the eyelids, the amount and weight of the skin covering the head and face, the orbital contents and the conformation of the skull.

C.   Glaucoma

Glaucoma is characterized by an elevation of intraocular pressure (IOP) which, when sustained, causes intraocular damage resulting in blindness. The elevated intraocular pressure occurs because the fluid cannot leave through the iridocorneal angle. Diagnosis and classification of glaucoma requires measurement of the IOP (tonometry) and examination of the iridocorneal angle (gonioscopy). Neither of these tests are part of a routine breed eye screening exam.

In this breed, primary glaucoma is associated with narrowed iridocorneal angles and various degrees of congenital angle malformations varying from mild to severe. Dysplastic pectinate ligaments and subsequent narrowed angles are similar to those described in the Basset and American and English Cocker Spaniels. The occurrence of glaucoma is related to the most severe abnormalities of the pectinate ligaments. The relationship between glaucoma development and the anomaly of the pectinate ligament is not clear.

References

1. Rubin LF: Inherited Eye Diseases in Purebred Dogs. Williams & Wilkins, Baltimore, 1989.

2. ACVO Genetics Committee, 1992 and/or Data from CERF All-Breeds Report, 1991.

3. Boeve' MH, Stades FC: Glaucoom bij hond en kat. Oversicht en retrospectieve evaluatie van 421 patienten I.Pathobiologischeachtergronden, indeling en raspredisposities. [Glaucoma in dogs and cats. Review and retrospective evaluation of 421 patients I. Pathobiological background, classification and breed predisposition]. Tijdschr Diergeneeskd 110: 219, 1985.

4. van der Linde-Sipman JS: Dysplasia of the pectinate ligament and primary glaucoma in the Bouvier des Flandres dog. Vet Pathol 24: 201, 1987.

BOXER

	DISORDER	INHERITANCE	REFERENCE	BREEDING ADVICE
A.	Distichiasis	Not defined	--	Breeder option
B.	Prolapsed gland of third eyelid	Not defined	--	Breeder option
C.	Corneal erosion	Not defined	1,2	Breeder option
D.	Non-pigmented third eyelid	Not defined	--	Breeder option

Description and Comments

This is a breed having a recognized multitude of disorders. There is no appreciable documentation of inherited traits. The incidence and problems of older boxers with ocular melanoma, corneal ulcerative keratitis, cataract, corneal exposure problems (ectropion) and corneal scarring from irritative problems (entropion and distichiasis) is rather accepted. Perhaps the major probable hereditary problems are entropion and corneal erosions, and the balance is due to poor conformation leading to globe exposure. Melanomas of the iris and ciliary body are answered by some other cause/effect.

A. Distichiasis

Eyelashes abnormally located in the eyelid margin which may cause ocular irritation. Distichiasis may occur at any time in the life of a dog. It is difficult to make a strong recommendation with regard to breeding dogs with this entity. The hereditary basis has not been established although it seems probable due to the high incidence in some breeds. Reducing the incidence is a logical goal. When diagnosed, distichiasis should be recorded; breeding discretion is advised.

B. Prolapse of the gland of the third eyelid

A protrusion of the tear gland associated with the third eyelid. The mode of inheritance of this disorder is unknown. The exposed gland may become irritated. The condition is commonly referred to as "cherry eye".

73

C.   Corneal erosion

A general group of corneal ulcerative conditions (e.g. erosions, indolent or persistent ulcers, epithelial bonding defects) is recognized as a common problem in older boxers (as well as other older animals). It has been commonly referred to as Boxer corneal ulceration. Animals that are affected are usually 7-8 years of age or older. The ulceration can be a very difficult lesion to heal, and it is often recurrent. The chronic form stimulates eventual scarring, with vascularization, fibrosis and pigmentation of the lesion site. The lesion can cause vision impairment.

D.   Unpigmented third eyelid

Some boxers have non-pigmented third eyelids from birth. Although the condition may be considered undesirable, the lack of pigment in no way affects normal function of the eye and does not represent a disease. Dogs with this condition alone (without any signs of irritation or disease which dictate consideration of removing the third eyelid) should not have the third eyelid removed.

References

1.   Gelatt KN, Samuelson DA: Recurrent corneal erosions and epithelial dystrophy in the boxer dog. J Am Anim Hosp Assoc 18:453, 1982.

2.   Roberts SR: Superficial indolent ulcer in the cornea of boxer dogs. J Small Anim Pract 6:111, 1965.

BRIARD

	DISORDER	INHERITANCE	REFERENCE	BREEDING ADVICE
A.	Cataract	Not defined	--	NO
B.	Progressive Retinal Atrophy	Not defined	1	NO
C.	Central Progressive Retinal Atrophy	Autosomal recessive	2	NO
D.	Stationary Night Blindness	Autosomal recessive	3,4,5	NO

Description and Comments

A.   Cataract

Lens opacity which may affect one or both eyes and may involve the lens partially or completely. In cases where cataracts are complete and affect both eyes, blindness results. The prudent approach is to assume cataracts to be hereditary except in cases known to be associated with trauma, other causes of ocular inflammation, specific metabolic diseases, persistent pupillary membranes, persistent hyaloid or nutritional deficiencies. The frequency and significance of cataracts in the breed is not known.

B.   Progressive Retinal Atrophy (PRA)

A degenerative disease of the retinal visual cells which progresses to blindness. This abnormality may be detected by electroretinogram before it is apparent clinically. In all breeds studied to date, PRA is recessively inherited. In the Briard, early fundus abnormalities usually appear after 4 years of age. The electroretinogram (ERG) shows marked functional abnormalities indicative of a progressive rod-cone degeneration. The age for early diagnosis by ERG has not been established but should be possible in dogs over 2 years of age.

C.   Central Progressive Retinal Atrophy (CPRA)

A progressive retinal degeneration in which photoreceptor death occurs secondary to disease of the underlying pigment epithelium. Progression is slow and some animals never lose vision. CPRA occurs in England, but is uncommon elsewhere.

In the Briard, the early lesions are seen first in the temporal tapetal fundus and progress to affect the posterior pole region at a later time; the eye lesions may initially be asymmetrical. The age of onset varies from young adults (> 17 months) to older animals. Many dogs have been found to be normal on repeated examinations before 5 years of age, only to develop clinical signs at a later age. The disease is inherited as a simple recessive trait. The ERG has not been reported to be a useful test for the early diagnosis of the disease.

D.   Congenital Stationary Night Blindness (CSNB)

A non-progressive retinal function defect characterized primarily by night blindness; day vision is normal to severely compromised. Ophthalmoscopic examination shows no abnormalities. The condition is detected by 5-6 weeks of age, after the postnatal maturation of the retina is completed. Nystagmus is present in some dogs, particularly in those having night blindness and severely compromised day vision. The ERG results are specific and diagnostic for the disorder. ERG testing is essential to distinguish this disorder from more central visual pathway defects which may appear clinically similar. The disease must also be distinguished from progressive retinal atrophy (PRA) from which it is distinct. Abnormalities in serum lipids (mild hypercholesterolemia) and elevated arachidonic acid have been noted in some animals. The significance of these findings is unknown.

References

1.   ACVO Genetics Committee, 1992 and/or Data from CERF All-Breeds Report, 1991.

2.   Bedford P: Retinal pigment epithelial dystrophy (CPRA): study of the disease in the briard. J Sm Anim Pract 25:129, 1984.

3.   Riis R and Aguirre G: The briard problem. Trans Amer Coll Vet Ophthalmol, 1983.

4.   Riis R and Siakotos A: Inherited lipid retinopathy in a dog breed. Suppl Invest Ophthalmol Vis Sci 30:308, 1989.

5.   Narfstrom K et al: The briard dog: a new animal model of congenital stationary night blindness. Brit J Ophthal 73:750, 1989.

BRITTANY SPANIEL

	DISORDER	INHERITANCE	REFERENCE	BREEDING ADVICE
A.	Cataract	Not defined	--	NO
B.	Lens luxation	Not defined	--	NO
C.	Progressive Retinal Atrophy	Not defined	--	NO

Description and Comments

A.   Cataract

Lens opacity which may affect one or both eyes and may involve the lens partially or completely. In cases where cataracts are complete and affect both eyes, blindness results. The prudent approach is to assume cataracts to be hereditary except in cases known to be associated with trauma, other causes of ocular inflammation, specific metabolic diseases, persistent pupillary membranes, persistent hyaloid or nutritional deficiencies. The exact frequency and significance of cataracts in the breed is not known, although it is probably low.

B.   Lens luxation

Partial (subluxated) or complete displacement of the lens from the normal anatomic site behind the pupil. Lens luxation not associated with trauma or inflammation is presumed to be inherited. Lens luxation may result in elevated intraocular pressure (glaucoma) causing vision impairment or blindness.

C.   Progressive Retinal Atrophy (PRA)

A degenerative disease of the retinal visual cells which progresses to blindness. This abnormality may be detected by electroretinogram before it is apparent clinically. In all breeds studied to date, PRA is recessively inherited. The exact frequency and significance of PRA in the breed is not known, although it is probably low.

Other Conditions Under Consideration

D.   Vitreous Degeneration

A liquefaction of the vitreous gel which may predispose to retinal detachment.

E.   Glaucoma

An elevation of intraocular pressure (IOP) which, when sustained, causes intraocular damage resulting in blindness. The elevated IOP occurs because the fluid cannot leave through the iridocorneal angle. Diagnosis and classification of glaucoma requires measurement of IOP (tonometry) and examination of the iridocorneal angle (gonioscopy). Neither of these tests are part of a routine breed eye screening exam.

References

There are no references providing detailed descriptions of hereditary conditions of the Brittany spaniel breed. The conditions listed above are generally recognized to exist in this breed, as evidenced by repeated references made in general texts.

1.   ACVO Genetics Committee, 1992 and/or Data from CERF All-Breeds Report, 1991.

BRUSSELS GRIFFON

	DISORDER	INHERITANCE	REFERENCES	BREEDING ADVICE
A.	Ectopic cilia	Not defined	1	Breeder option
B.	Cataract	Not defined	1	NO
C.	Progressive Retinal Atrophy	Not defined	1	NO

Description and Comments

A.   Ectopic cilia

Hair emerging through the eyelid conjunctiva. Ectopic cilia occur more frequently in younger dogs and cause discomfort and corneal disease.

B.   Cataract

Lens opacity which may affect one or both eyes and may involve the lens partially or completely. In cases where cataracts are complete and affect both eyes, blindness results. The prudent approach is to assume cataracts to be hereditary except in cases known to be associated with trauma, other causes of ocular inflammation, specific metabolic diseases, persistent pupillary membrane, persistent hyaloid or nutritional deficiencies.

C.   Progressive Retinal Atrophy (PRA)

A degenerative disease of the retinal visual cells which progresses to blindness. This abnormality may be detected by electroretinogram before it is apparent clinically. In all breeds studied to date, PRA is recessively inherited.

References

There are no references providing detailed descriptions of hereditary ocular conditions of the Brussels Griffon breed. The conditions listed above are generally recognized to exist in this breed, as evidenced by repeated references made in general texts.

1.   ACVO Genetics Committee, 1992 and/or Data from CERF All-Breeds Report, 1991.

BULLDOG

	DISORDER	INHERITANCE	REFERENCE	BREEDING ADVICE
A.	Entropion	Not defined	1	Breeder option
B.	Ectropion	Not defined	2	Breeder option
C.	Distichiasis	Not defined	1	Breeder option
D.	Ectopic cilia	Not defined	1	Breeder option
E.	Prolapsed gland of third eyelid	Not defined	3	Breeder option
F.	Dry eye	Not defined	4	Breeder option

Description and Comments

A.   Entropion

A conformational defect resulting in an "in-rolling" of one or more of the eyelids which may cause ocular irritation. It is likely that entropion is influenced by several genes (polygenic), defining the skin and other structures which make up the eyelids, the amount and weight of the skin covering the head and face, the orbital contents, and the conformation of the skull.

B.   Ectropion

A conformational defect resulting in eversion of the eyelids which may cause ocular irritation due to exposure. It is likely that ectropion is influenced by several genes (polygenic) defining the skin and other structures which make up the eyelids, the amount and weight of the skin covering the head and face, the orbital contents and the conformation of the skull.

In the Bulldog, ectropion is associated with an exceptionally large palpebral fissure and laxity of the canthal structures. Central lower lid ectropion is often associated with entropion of the adjacent lid. This causes severe ocular irritation.

C.   Distichiasis

Eyelashes abnormally located in the eyelid margin which may cause ocular irritation. Distichiasis may occur at any time in the life of a dog. It is difficult to make a strong recommendation with regard to breeding dogs with this entity. The hereditary basis has not been established although it seems probable due to the high incidence in some breeds. Reducing the incidence is a logical goal. When diagnosed, distichiasis should be recorded; breeding discretion is advised.

D.   Ectopic cilia

Hair emerging through the eyelid conjunctiva. Ectopic cilia occur more frequently in younger dogs and cause discomfort and corneal disease.

E.   Prolapse of the gland of the third eyelid

Protrusion of the tear gland associated with the third eyelid. The mode of inheritance of this disorder is unknown. The exposed gland may become irritated. Commonly referred to as "cherry eye".

F.   Dry eye

An abnormality of the tear film, most commonly a deficiency of the aqueous portion, although the mucin and/or lipid layers may be affected; results in ocular irritation and/or vision impairment.

Other Conditions Under Consideration

G.   Retinal Dysplasia - folds

Abnormal development of the retina present at birth and recognized to have three forms:

      1) Retinal dysplasia - **folds**: linear, triangular, curved or curvilinear foci of retinal folding that may be single or multiple.
      2) Retinal dysplasia - **geographic**: any irregularly shaped area of abnormal retinal development, representing changes not accountable by simple folding.
      3) Retinal dysplasia - **detachment**: either of the above described forms of retinal dysplasia associated with separation (detachment) of the retina.

The two latter forms are associated with vision impairment or blindness. Retinal dysplasia is known to be inherited in many breeds. The genetic relationship between the three forms of the disease is not known for all breeds.

82

References

1. ACVO Genetics Committee, 1992 and/or Data from CERF All-Breeds Report, 1991.

2. Priester WA: Congenital ocular defects in cattle, horses, cats and dogs. J Am Vet Med Assoc 160:1504, 1972.

3. Barnett KC: Comparative aspects of canine hereditary eye disease. Adv Vet Sci Comp Med 20:39, 1976.

4. Kaswan RL et al: Immunological evaluation of 62 dogs with keratoconjunctivitis sicca. Trans Am Coll Vet Ophthalmol, 1983, p207.

BULLMASTIFF

	DISORDER	INHERITANCE	REFERENCE	BREEDING ADVICE
A.	Entropion	Not defined	1	Breeder option
B.	Distichiasis	Not defined	1	Breeder option
C.	Persistent pupillary membrane	Not defined	1	Breeder option
D.	Retinal dysplasia	Not defined	1	Breeder option
E.	Glaucoma	Not defined	1	NO

Description and Comments

A.   Entropion

A conformational defect resulting in an "in-rolling" of one or more of the eyelids which may cause ocular irritation. It is likely that entropion is influenced by several genes (polygenic) defining the skin and other structures which make up the eyelids, the amount and weight of the skin covering the head and face, the orbital contents and the conformation of the skull.

In this breed, the palpebral fissures may become vertical and/or shaped like a "pagoda". Entropion in the Bullmastiff generally requires surgical correction.

B.   Distichiasis

Eyelashes abnormally located in the eyelid margin which may cause ocular irritation. Distichiasis may occur at any time in the life of a dog. It is difficult to make a strong recommendation with regard to breeding dogs with this entity. The hereditary basis has not been established although it seems probable due to the high incidence in some breeds. Reducing the incidence is a logical goal. When diagnosed, distichiasis should be recorded. Breeding discretion is advised.

C. Persistent pupillary membrane (PPM)

Persistent blood vessel remnants in the anterior chamber of the eye which fail to regress normally in the neonatal period. These strands may bridge from iris to iris, iris to cornea, iris to lens, or form sheets of tissue in the anterior chamber. The last three forms pose the greatest threat to vision and when severe, vision impairment or blindness may occur.

D. Retinal dysplasia

Abnormal development of the retina present at birth and recognized to have three forms:

1) Retinal dysplasia - **folds**: linear, triangular, curved or curvilinear foci of retinal folding that may be single or multiple.
2) Retinal dysplasia - **geographic**: any irregularly shaped area of abnormal retinal development representing changes not accountable by simple folding.
3) Retinal dysplasia - **detachment**: either of the above described forms of retinal dysplasia associated with separation (detachment) of the retina.

The two latter forms are associated with vision impairment or blindness. Retinal dysplasia is known to be inherited in many breeds. The genetic relationship between the three forms of the disease is not known for all breeds.

The fold form is the type observed in the Bullmastiff.

E. Glaucoma

Glaucoma is characterized by an elevation of intraocular pressure (IOP) which, when sustained, causes intraocular damage resulting in blindness. The elevated IOP occurs because the fluid cannot leave through the iridocorneal angle. Diagnosis and classification of glaucoma requires measurement of the IOP (tonometry) and examination of the iridocorneal angle (gonioscopy). Neither of these tests are part of a routine breed eye screening exam.

References

There are no references providing detailed descriptions of hereditary ocular conditions of the Bullmastiff breed. The conditions listed above are generally recognized to exist in this breed, as evidenced by repeated references made in general texts.

1. ACVO Genetics Committee, 1992 and/or Data from CERF All-Breeds Report, 1991.

BULL TERRIER

	DISORDER	INHERITANCE	REFERENCE	BREEDING ADVICE
A.	Entropion	Not defined	1,2	Breeder option
B.	Ectropion	Not defined	1	Breeder option

Description and Comments

A.   Entropion

A conformational defect resulting in "in-rolling" of one or more of the eyelids which may cause ocular irritation. It is likely that entropion is influenced by several genes (polygenic), defining the skin and other structures which make up the eyelids, the amount and weight of the skin covering the head and face, the orbital contents and the conformation of the skull.

B.   Ectropion

A conformational defect resulting in eversion of the eyelids, which may cause ocular irritation due to exposure. It is likely that ectropion is influenced by several genes (polygenic), defining the skin and other structures which make up the eyelids, the amount and weight of the skin covering the head and face, the orbital contents and the conformation of the skull. Ectropion in the Bull Terrier is usually mild and rarely requires surgical correction.

References

1.   ACVO Genetics Committee, 1992 and/or Data from CERF All-Breeds Report, 1991.

2.   Johnston DE, Cox B: The incidence in purebred dogs in Australia of abnormalities that may be inherited. Aust Vet J 46: 465, 1970.

CAIRN TERRIER

	DISORDER	INHERITANCE	REFERENCE	BREEDING ADVICE
A.	Cataract	Not defined	1	NO
B.	Glaucoma (pigmentary)	Not defined	2	NO

Description and Comments

A.   Cataract

Lens opacity which may affect one or both eyes and may involve the lens partially or completely. In cases where cataracts are complete and affect both eyes, blindness results. The prudent approach is to assume cataracts to be hereditary except in cases known to be associated with trauma, other causes of ocular inflammation, specific metabolic diseases, persistent pupillary membranes, persistent hyaloid or nutritional deficiencies.

B.   Pigmentary glaucoma

Glaucoma is characterized by an elevation of intraocular pressure (IOP) which, when sustained, causes intraocular damage resulting in blindness. The elevated IOP occurs because the fluid cannot leave through the iridocorneal angle. Diagnosis and classification of glaucoma requires measurement of the IOP (tonometry) and examination of the iridocorneal angle (gonioscopy). Neither of these tests are part of a routine breed eye screening exam.

References

1.   ACVO Genetics Committee, 1992 and/or CERF All-Breeds Report, 1991.

2.   Covitz D, Barthold S, Dithers R, Riis R: "Pigmentary glaucoma" in the Cairn terrier. Trans Am Coll Vet Ophthalmol, 15: 245, 1984.

3.   Petersen-Jones SM: Abnormal ocular pigment deposition associated with glaucoma in the Cairn terrier. J Small Anim Pract 32: 19, 1991.

CAVALIER KING CHARLES SPANIEL

	DISORDER	INHERITANCE	REFERENCE	BREEDING ADVICE
A.	Microphthalmia	Not defined	1	NO
B.	Distichiasis	Not defined	2	Breeder option
C.	Entropion	Not defined	2	Breeder option
D.	Corneal dystrophy	Not defined	3	Breeder option
E.	Exposure keratopathy/ macroblepharon	Not defined	2	Breeder option
F.	Cataract	Not defined	2	NO
G.	Retinal dysplasia - folds	Not defined	2	Breeder option
	Retinal dysplasia - geographic/detached	Not defined	2	NO

Description and Comments

A.   Microphthalmia/multiple congenital ocular defects

Microphthalmia is a congenital defect characterized by a small eye with associated defects of the cornea, anterior chamber, lens and/or retina.

B.   Distichiasis

Eyelashes abnormally located in the eyelid margin which may cause ocular irritation. Distichiasis may occur at any time in the life of a dog. It is difficult to make a strong recommendation with regard to breeding dogs with this entity. The hereditary basis has not been established, although it seems probable due to the high incidence in some breeds. Reducing the incidence is a logical goal. When diagnosed, distichiasis should be recorded; breeding discretion is advised.

C.   Entropion

A conformational defect resulting in an "in-rolling" of one or more of the eyelids which may cause ocular irritation. It is likely that entropion is influenced by several genes (polygenic), defining the skin and other structures which make up the eyelids, the amount and weight of the skin covering the head and face, the orbital contents, and the conformation of the skull.

In this breed, the medial aspect of the eyelid is most frequently affected and tearing is the most prominent sign.

D.   Corneal dystrophy

A non-inflammatory corneal opacity (white to gray) present in one or more of the corneal layers. Corneal dystrophy implies a probable inherited basis and is usually bilateral.

E.   Exposure keratopathy / macroblepharon

A corneal disease involving all or part of the cornea, resulting from inadequate blinking. This results from a combination of anatomic features including shallow orbits, exophthalmos, macroblepharon and lagophthalmos.

F.   Cataract

Lens opacity which may affect one or both eyes and may involve the lens partially or completely. In cases where cataracts are complete and affect both eyes, blindness results. The prudent approach is to assume cataracts to be hereditary except in cases known to be associated with trauma, other causes of ocular inflammation, specific metabolic diseases, persistent pupillary membranes, persistent hyaloid or nutritional deficiencies.

G.   Multifocal retinal dysplasia

Abnormal development of the retina present at birth and recognized to have three forms:

1) Retinal dysplasia - **folds**: linear, triangular, curved or curvilinear foci of retinal folding that may be single or multiple.
2) Retinal dysplasia - **geographic**: any irregularly shaped area of abnormal retinal development, representing changes not accountable by simple folding.
3) Retinal dysplasia - **detachment**: either of the above described forms of retinal dysplasia associated with separation (detachment) of the retina.

The two latter forms are associated with vision impairment or blindness. Retinal dysplasia is known to be inherited in many breeds. The genetic relationship between the three forms of the disease is not known for all breeds.

References

1.   Narfstrom K et al: Posterior lenticonus, cataracts and microphthalmia: congenital defects in the Cavalier King Charles spaniel. J Small Anim Pract 25:669, 1984.

2.   ACVO Genetics Committee, 1992 and/or Data from CERF All-Breeds Report, 1991.

3.   Crispin SM: Crystalline stromal dystrophy in the Cavalier King Charles spaniel. Trans Am Coll Vet Ophthalmol 1986, p.18.

CHESAPEAKE BAY RETRIEVER

	DISORDER	INHERITANCE	REFERENCE	BREEDING ADVICE
A.	Entropion	Not defined	--	Breeder option
B.	Distichiasis	Not defined	1	Breeder option
C.	Cataract	Not defined	2	NO
D.	Progressive retinal atrophy	Not defined	1	NO
E.	Retinal dysplasia - folds	Not defined	1	NO
F.	Retinal dysplasia - geographic	Not defined	1	NO

Description and Comments

A. Entropion

A conformational defect resulting in "in-rolling" of one or more of the eyelids which may cause ocular irritation. It is likely that entropion is influenced by several genes (polygenic), defining the skin and other structures which make up the eyelids, the amount and weight of the skin covering the head and face, the orbital contents and the conformation of the skull. Selection should be directed against entropion and toward a head conformation that minimizes or eliminates the likelihood of the defect.

B. Distichiasis

Eyelashes abnormally located in the eyelid margin which may cause ocular irritation. Distichiasis may occur at any time in the life of a dog. It is difficult to make a strong recommendation with regard to breeding dogs with this entity. The hereditary basis has not been established, although it seems probable due to the high incidence in some breeds. Reducing the incidence is a logical goal. When diagnosed, distichiasis should be recorded; breeding discretion is advised.

C.   Cataract

Lens opacity which may affect one or both eyes and may involve the lens partially or completely. In cases where cataracts are complete and affect both eyes, blindness results. The prudent approach is to assume cataracts to be hereditary except in cases known to be associated with trauma, other causes of ocular inflammation, specific metabolic diseases, persistent pupillary membranes, persistent hyaloid or nutritional deficiencies.

Hereditary cataracts have been described in the breed and affect the young adult dog. They appear as posterior cortical, axial, triangular opacities and the Y suture tips can be affected in both the anterior and posterior cortices. Extension of the cataract into the posterior cortex and progression to impair vision can occur. An autosomal dominant inheritance with incomplete penetrance has been proposed; however, the genetics have not been completely defined and additional studies will be required.

D.   Progressive Retinal Atrophy (PRA)

A degenerative disease of the retinal visual cells which progresses to blindness. This abnormality may be detected by electroretinogram before it is apparent clinically. In all breeds studied to date, PRA is recessively inherited.

Ophthalmoscopic abnormalities characteristic of mid-stage disease are found in dogs between 8-12 months of age. The lesions are progressive and end-stage lesions are evident by 2-3 years of age. Other affected dogs have similar ophthalmoscopic lesions, but these are present at a later age (4-7 years). It is possible that two different types of PRA (early onset and late onset) are present in the breed; such a situation occurs in the Norwegian Elkhound. The age for early diagnosis by ERG has not been definitively established for the breed.

E.   Retinal Dysplasia - Folds
F.   Retinal Dysplasia - Geographic

Abnormal development of the retina present at birth and recognized to have three forms:

   1) Retinal dysplasia - **folds**: linear, triangular, curved or curvilinear foci of retinal folding that may be single or multiple.
   2) Retinal dysplasia - **geographic**: any irregularly shaped area of abnormal retinal development, representing changes not accountable by simple folding.
   3) Retinal dysplasia - **detachment**: either of the above described forms of retinal dysplasia associated with separation (detachment) of the retina.

The two latter forms are associated with vision impairment or blindness. Retinal dysplasia is known to be inherited in many breeds. The genetic relationship between the three forms of the disease is not known for all breeds.

References

1. ACVO Genetics Committee, 1992 and/or Data from CERF All-Breeds Report, 1991.

2. Gelatt KN et al: Cataracts in Chesapeake Bay retrievers. J Am Vet Med Assoc 175:1176, 1979.

3. Acland GM and Aguirre GD: Retinal degeneration in the dog. IV. Early retinal degeneration (*erd*) in Norwegian Elkhounds. Exp Eye Res 44:491, 1987.

CHIHUAHUA

	DISORDER	INHERITANCE	REFERENCE	BREEDING ADVICE
A.	Endothelial dystrophy	Not defined	1	NO
B.	Progressive Retinal Atrophy	Not defined	2	NO

Description and Comments

A. Corneal endothelial dystrophy

A primary degenerative endothelial disease leading to progressive and permanent corneal edema. It is not known if this disease is an inherited disorder. There is no sex predilection. The condition is observed in older dogs, 6 to 13 years of age with a mean of 9.5 years.

The corneal edema starts asymptomatically in the dorsal temporal corneal quadrant of one eye and slowly progresses medially, eventually involving the entire cornea. Typically, it eventually becomes bilateral. In the later stages, discomfort, intracorneal bullae with subsequent ulceration and keratoconus may develop. Histologically, the primary endothelial disease appears slightly different than the clinically similar appearing disorder of the Boston Terrier.

B. Progressive Retinal Atrophy (PRA)

A degenerative disease of the retinal visual cells which progresses to blindness. This abnormality may be detected by electroretinogram before it is apparent clinically. In all breeds studied to date, PRA is recessively inherited.

Conditions Under Consideration

C. Lens luxation

Partial or complete displacement of the lens from the normal anatomic site. Lens luxation not associated with trauma or inflammation is presumed to be inherited and may cause visual impairment or blindness.

94

References

1. Martin CL, Dice PF: Corneal endothelial dystrophy in the dog. J Am Anim Hosp Assoc 18:327, 1982.

2. ACVO Genetics Committee, 1992 and/or Data from CERF All-Breeds Report, 1991.

CHOW CHOW

	DISORDER	INHERITANCE	REFERENCE	BREEDING ADVICE
A.	Entropion	Not defined	1	Breeder option
B.	Glaucoma	Not defined	1	NO
C.	Progressive Retinal Atrophy	Not defined	1	NO
D.	Persistent pupillary membrane	Not defined	1	NO

DESCRIPTION AND COMMENTS

A. Entropion

A conformational defect resulting in an "in-rolling" of one or more of the eyelids which may cause ocular irritation. It is likely that entropion is influenced by several genes (polygenic), defining the skin and other structures which make up the eyelids, the amount and weight of the skin covering the head and face, the orbital contents, and the conformation of the skull.

Entropion in the Chow Chow has been observed for decades and is definitely related to the amount of skin covering the head and face. Because of the conformation admired by both fanciers and the judges, it is doubtful that we will see a significant change in the incidence of entropion as folds are, in many cases, desired by these individuals. Entropion requires surgical correction in the Chow Chow to return comfort and decrease chances for vision loss.

B. Glaucoma

Glaucoma is characterized by an elevation of intraocular pressure which when sustained causes intraocular damage resulting in blindness. The elevated intraocular pressure occurs because the fluid cannot leave through the iridocorneal angle. Diagnosis and classification of glaucoma requires measurement of the intraocular pressure (tonometry) and examination of the iridocorneal angle (gonioscopy). Neither of these tests are part of a routine breed eye screening exam.

Age of onset in the Chow Chow appears to be anywhere between 3-6 years of age and has been observed as a bilateral condition. Gonioscopy has evidenced extremely narrow iridocorneal angles and in many regions no evidence of trabecular meshwork.

C.   Progressive Retinal Atrophy (PRA)

A degenerative disease of the retinal visual cells which progresses to blindness. This abnormality may be detected by electroretinogram before it is apparent clinically. In all breeds studied to date, PRA is recessively inherited.

In the United States, PRA is not common in the Chow Chow but has been observed.

D.   Persistent pupillary membrane (PPM)

Persistent blood vessel remnants in the anterior chamber of the eye which fail to regress normally in the neonatal period. These strands may bridge from iris to iris, iris to cornea, iris to lens, or form sheets of tissue in the anterior chamber. The last three forms pose the greatest threat to vision and when severe, vision impairment or blindness may occur.

Major PPM's have been observed in this breed. Many ophthalmologists have observed puppies so severely affected that they are temporarily or permanently blind. The blindness is due to adherence of the membranes to the cornea and/or lens.

References

There are no references providing detailed descriptions of hereditary ocular conditions of the Chow Chow breed. The conditions listed above are generally recognized to exist in this breed, as evidenced by repeated references made in general texts.

1.   ACVO Genetics Committee, 1992 and/or Data from CERF All-Breeds Report, 1991.

CLUMBER SPANIEL

	DISORDER	INHERITANCE	REFERENCE	BREEDING ADVICE
A.	Ectropion	Not defined	1	Breeder option
B.	Entropion	Not defined	2	Breeder option
C.	Macroblepharon	Not defined	1	Breeder option

Description and Comments

A.   Ectropion

A conformational defect resulting in eversion of the eyelids, which may cause ocular irritation. It is likely that ectropion is influenced by several genes (polygenic), defining the skin and other structures which make up the eyelids, the amount and weight of the skin covering the head and face, the orbital contents and the conformation of the skull.

B.   Entropion

A conformational defect resulting in "in-rolling" of one or more of the eyelids, which may cause ocular irritation. It is likely that entropion is influenced by several genes (polygenic), defining the skin and other structures which make up the eyelids, the amount and weight of the skin covering the head and face, the orbital contents and the conformation of the skull.

C.   Macroblepharon

Abnormally large eyelid opening; may lead to secondary conditions associated with corneal exposure.

References

1.   ACVO Genetics Committee, 1992 and/or Data from CERF All-Breeds Report, 1991.

2.   Hodgman SFJ: Abnormalities and defects in pedigree dogs. I. An investigation into the existence of abnormalities in pedigree dogs in the British Isles. J Small Anim Pract 4:447, 1963.

(AMERICAN) COCKER SPANIEL

The official breed name is Cocker Spaniel. The designation "American" has been used to avoid confusion and emphasize the distinction from the English Cocker Spaniel breed.

	DISORDER	INHERITANCE	REFERENCE	BREEDING ADVICE
A.	Progressive Retinal Atrophy	Autosomal recessive	1,2	NO
B.	Retinal dysplasia	Not defined		
	- focal		3	Breeder option
	- geographic/detachment		4	NO
C.	Cataract			
	1. Cortical	Autosomal recessive	5-9	NO
	2. Other types	Not defined	--	See comments
D.	Corneal dystrophy	Not defined	4	Breeder option
E.	Persistent pupillary membrane	Not defined	--	Breeder option
F.	Glaucoma	Not defined	10-13	NO
G.	Dry eye	Not defined	--	Breeder option
H.	Imperforate lacrimal punctum	Not defined	--	Breeder option
I.	Prolapsed gland of third eyelid	Not defined	--	Breeder option
J.	Ectropion	Not defined	--	Breeder option
K.	Distichiasis	Not defined	14,15	Breeder option

Description and Comments

A.   Progressive Retinal Atrophy (PRA)

A degenerative disease of the retinal visual cells which progresses to blindness. This abnormality may be detected by electroretinogram before it is apparent clinically. In all breeds studied to date, PRA is recessively inherited.

B.   Retinal dysplasia

Abnormal development of the retina present at birth and recognized to have three forms:

1) Retinal dysplasia - **folds**: linear, triangular, curved or curvilinear foci of retinal folding that may be single or multiple.
2) Retinal dysplasia - **geographic**: any irregularly shaped area of abnormal retinal development, representing changes not accountable by simple folding.
3) Retinal dysplasia - **detachment**: either of the above described forms of retinal dysplasia associated with separation (detachment) of the retina.

The two latter forms are associated with vision impairment or blindness. Retinal dysplasia is known to be inherited in many breeds. The genetic relationship between the three forms of the disease is not known for all breeds.

C.   Cataract

Lens opacity which may affect one or both eyes and may involve the lens partially or completely. In cases where cataracts are complete and affect both eyes, blindness results. The prudent approach is to assume cataracts to be hereditary except in cases known to be associated with trauma, other causes of ocular inflammation, specific metabolic diseases, persistent pupillary membranes, persistent hyaloid or nutritional deficiencies.

D.   Corneal dystrophy

A non-inflammatory corneal opacity (white to gray) present in one or more of the corneal layers; usually inherited and bilateral.

E.   Persistent pupillary membranes (PPM)

Persistent blood vessel remnants in the anterior chamber of the eye which fail to regress normally in the neonatal period. These strands may bridge from iris to iris, iris to cornea, iris to lens, or form sheets of tissue in the anterior chamber. The last three forms pose the greatest threat to vision and when severe, vision impairment or blindness may occur.

F. Glaucoma

An elevation of intraocular pressure (IOP) which, when sustained, causes intraocular damage resulting in blindness. The elevated IOP occurs because the fluid cannot leave through the iridocorneal angle. Diagnosis and classification of glaucoma requires measurement of IOP (tonometry) and examination of the iridocorneal angle (gonioscopy). Neither of these tests are part of a routine breed eye screening exam.

G. Dry eye

An abnormality of the tear film, most commonly a deficiency of the aqueous portion, although the mucin and/or lipid layers may be affected; results in ocular irritation and/or vision impairment.

H. Imperforate lacrimal punctum

A developmental anomaly resulting in failure of opening of the lacrimal duct adjacent to the eye. The lower punctum is more frequently affected. This defect usually results in epiphora, an overflow of tears onto the face.

I. Prolapsed gland of the third eyelid

Protrusion of the tear gland associated with the third eyelid. The mode of inheritance of this disorder is unknown. The exposed gland may become irritated. Commonly referred to as "cherry eye".

J. Ectropion

A conformational defect resulting in eversion of the eyelids, which may cause ocular irritation due to exposure. It is likely that ectropion is influenced by several genes (polygenic) defining the skin and other structures which make up the eyelids, the amount and weight of the skin covering the head and face, the orbital contents and the conformation of the skull.

K. Distichiasis

Eyelashes abnormally located in the eyelid margin which may cause ocular irritation. Distichiasis may occur at any time in the life of a dog. It is difficult to make a strong recommendation with regard to breeding dogs with this entity. The hereditary basis has not been established although it seems probable due to the high incidence in some breeds. Reducing the incidence is a logical goal. When diagnosed, distichiasis should be recorded; breeding discretion is advised.

References

1. Barnett KC: Canine retinopathies III. Other breeds. J Small Anim Pract 6:185, 1965.

2. Aguirre G, Acland G: Variation in retinal degeneration phenotype inherited at the PRCD locus. Exp Eye Res 46:663, 1988.

3. MacMillan AD, Lipton DE: Heritability of multifocal retinal dysplasia in the American Cocker spaniel. J Am Vet Med Assoc 172:568, 1978.

4. ACVO Genetics Committee, 1992 and/or Data from CERF All-Breeds Report, 1991.

5. Barnett KC: Comparative aspects of canine hereditary eye disease. Adv Vet Sci Comp Med 20:39, 1976.

6. Gelatt KN: Lens and cataract formation in the dog. Comp Cont Ed 1:175, 1979.

7. Yakely WL: Familial cataracts in the American Cocker spaniel. J Am Anim Hosp Assoc 7:127, 1971.

8. Yakely WL: Cataracts in the American Cocker spaniel. Proc Am Coll Vet Ophthalmol 6:27, 1975.

9. Yakely WL: A study of inheritability of cataracts in the American Cocker spaniel. J Am Vet Med Assoc 172:814, 1978.

10. Brooks DE et al: Canine glaucoma: Pathogenesis, diagnosis and treatment. Comp Cont Ed 5:292, 1983.

11. Gelatt KN: Animal models for glaucoma. Invest Ophthalmol Vis Sci 6:592, 1977.

12. Lovekin LG et al: Clinicopathologic changes in primary glaucoma in the Cocker spaniel. Am J Vet Res 29:379, 1978.

13. Peiffer RL: Animal models of glaucoma. ILAR News 26:10, 1983.

14. Bedford PGC: The treatment of canine distichiasis by the method of partial tarsal plate excision. J Am Anim Hosp Assoc 15:59, 1979.

15. Lavach JD: Diseases of the eyelids (Part II). Comp Cont Ed 1: 485, 1979.

COLLIE

	DISORDER	INHERITANCE	REFERENCE	BREEDING ADVICE
A.	Microphthalmia	Not defined	1,2	NO
B.	Entropion	Not defined	3	Breeder option
C.	Distichiasis	Not defined	3	Breeder option
D.	Persistent pupillary membrane	Not defined	3	Breeder option
E.	Progressive Retinal Atrophy			
	1. Rod/cone dysplasia	Autosomal recessive	4	NO
	2. Rod/cone degeneration	Not defined	3	NO
F.	Choroidal hypoplasia +/- coloboma +/- retinal detachment	Not defined	5	NO
G.	Retinal dysplasia - folds	Not defined	3	Breeder option

Description and Comments

A.   Microphthalmia

A developmental anomaly in which the eyeball is abnormally small. This is often associated with other ocular malformations, including defects of the cornea, anterior chamber, lens and/or retina.

An association has been made between partial albinism, multiple ocular defects (especially microphthalmia) and deafness in a number of canine breeds including the Collie. From these reports it appears that a predominantly white hair coat is associated with a higher incidence of ocular defects.

B.   Entropion

A conformational defect resulting in an "in-rolling" of one or more of the eyelids which may cause ocular irritation. It is likely that entropion is influenced by several genes (polygenic), defining the skin and other structures which make up the eyelids, the amount and weight of the skin covering the head and face, the orbital contents, and the conformation of the skull.

C.   Distichiasis

Eyelashes abnormally located in the eyelid margin which may cause ocular irritation. Distichiasis may occur at any time. The hereditary basis has not been established although it seems probable due to the high incidence in some breeds. Reducing the incidence is a logical goal. In the collie, because there is significant clinical disease associated with the abnormal hairs, breeding should be discouraged.

D.   Persistent pupillary membranes

Persistent blood vessel remnants in the anterior chamber of the eye which fail to regress normally in the neonatal period. These strands may bridge from iris to iris, iris to cornea, iris to lens, or form sheets of tissue in the anterior chamber. The last three forms pose the greatest threat to vision and when severe, vision impairment or blindness may occur.

E.   Progressive Retinal Atrophy (PRA)

A degenerative disease of the retinal visual cells which progresses to blindness. This abnormality may be detected by electroretinogram before it is apparent clinically. In all breeds studied to date, PRA is recessively inherited.

In the Collie, two forms of this condition exist. In rod/cone dysplasia, the visual cells fail to develop normally and degenerate within the first year of life, resulting in blindness. In rod/cone degeneration (which occurs much less commonly), the visual cells develop normally and then undergo degeneration, with blindness occurring in the adult dog (age 5-7 years).

F.   Choroidal hypoplasia / Coloboma / Retinal detachment

A spectrum of malformations present at birth and ranging from inadequate development of the choroid (choroidal hypoplasia) to defects of the choroid, retina, or optic nerve (coloboma) to complete retinal detachment. Mildly affected animals will have no detectable vision deficit.

This disorder is collectively referred to as Collie Eye Anomaly. Although there is a lack of scientific evidence, it is believed that the incidence and severity of this entity was decreased by breeding only "mildly affected" Collies. At this time, the Genetics Committee of the ACVO recommends against breeding Collies with any form of the Collie Eye anomaly.

G.   Retinal dysplasia

Abnormal development of the retina present at birth and recognized to have three forms:

1) Retinal dysplasia - **folds**: linear, triangular, curved or curvilinear foci of retinal folding that may be single or multiple.
2) Retinal dysplasia - **geographic**: any irregularly shaped area of abnormal retinal development, representing changes not accountable by simple folding.
3) Retinal dysplasia - **detachment**: either of the above described forms of retinal dysplasia associated with separation (detachment) of the retina.

The two latter forms are associated with vision impairment or blindness. Retinal dysplasia is known to be inherited in many breeds. The genetic relationship between the three forms of the disease is not known for all breeds.

Other Conditions Under Consideration

H.   Proliferative keratoconjunctivitis

An acquired condition characterized by a progressive, pink, fleshy mass involving the cornea, raised bands of inflammatory tissue on the anterior aspect of the nictitating membrane, and conjunctivitis. The condition is most likely immune-mediated but affects Collies more frequently than other breeds.

References

1.   Gwin RM et al: Multiple ocular defects associated with partial albinism and deafness in the dog. J Am Anim Hosp Assoc 17:401, 1981.

2.   Bertram T, Coiqnoul F, Cheville N: Ocular dysgenesis in Australian shepherd dogs. J Am Anim Hosp Assoc 20:177, 1984.

3.   ACVO Genetics Committee, 1992 and/or Data from CERF All-Breeds Report, 1991.

4.   Wolf ED et al: Rod-cone dysplasia in the collie. J Am Vet Med Assoc 173:1331, 1978.

5.   Yakely WL et al: Genetic transmission of an ocular fundus anomaly in Collies. J Am Vet Med Assoc 152:457, 1968.

6.   Blogg RJ: Proliferative keratoconjunctivitis in the Collie. Trans Am Coll of Vet Ophthalmol 8:89, 1977.

7.   Smith JS: Infiltrative corneal lesions resembling fibrous histiocytoma. J Am Vet Med Assoc 169:722, 1976.

COONHOUND (Black and Tan)

	DISORDER	INHERITANCE	REFERENCE	BREEDING ADVICE
A.	Entropion	Not defined	1	NO
B.	Ectropion	Not defined	1	Breeder option

Description and Comments

A.   Entropion

A conformational defect resulting in an "in-rolling" of one or more of the eyelids which may cause ocular irritation. It is likely that entropion is influenced by several genes (polygenic), defining the skin and other structures which make up the eyelids, the amount and weight of the skin covering the head and face, the orbital contents, and the conformation of the skull. In this breed, entropion is associated with an exceptionally large palpebral fissure.

B.   Ectropion

A conformational defect resulting in eversion of the eyelids which may cause ocular irritation. It is likely that ectropion is influenced by several genes (polygenic) defining the skin and other structures which make up the eyelids, the amount and weight of the skin covering the head and face, the orbital contents and the conformation of the skull.

References

There are no references providing detailed descriptions of hereditary ocular conditions of the Black and Tan Coonhound breed. The conditions listed above are generally recognized to exist in this breed, as evidenced by repeated references made in general texts.

1.   ACVO Genetics Committee, 1992 and/or Data from CERF All-Breeds Report, 1991.

CURLY-COATED RETRIEVER

	DISORDER	INHERITANCE	REFERENCE	BREEDING ADVICE
A.	Entropion	Not defined	1	Breeder option
B.	Ectropion	Not defined	2	Breeder option
C.	Cataract			
	1. Anterior subcapsular	Not defined	1	NO
	2. Posterior subcapsular	Not defined	1,3	NO
D.	Progressive Retinal Atrophy	Not defined	1,3	NO

Description and Comments

A.   Entropion

A conformational defect resulting in an "in-rolling" of one or more of the eyelids which may cause ocular irritation. It is likely that entropion is influenced by several genes (polygenic), defining the skin and other structures which make up the eyelids, the amount and weight of the skin covering the head and face, the orbital contents, and the conformation of the skull.

B.   Ectropion

A conformational defect resulting in eversion of the eyelids which may cause ocular irritation due to exposure. It is likely that ectropion is influenced by several genes (polygenic) defining the skin and other structures which make up the eyelids, the amount and weight of the skin covering the head and face, the orbital contents and the conformation of the skull.

C.   Cataract

Lens opacity which may affect one or both eyes and may involve the lens partially or completely. In cases where cataracts are complete and affect both eyes, blindness results. The prudent approach is to assume cataracts to be hereditary except in cases known to be associated with trauma, other causes of ocular inflammation, specific metabolic diseases, persistent pupillary membranes, persistent hyaloid or nutritional deficiencies.

1.   Anterior cortical subcapsular cataract: Anterior subcapsular striate cortical cataracts usually occur bilaterally, slowly progress and usually occur between 5-8 years of age.

2.   Posterior subcapsular cataract: Posterior polar subcapsular opacities occur at 2-4 years of age and progress slowly.

C.   Progressive Retinal Atrophy (PRA)

A degenerative disease of the retinal visual cells which progresses to blindness. This abnormality may be detected by electroretinogram before it is apparent clinically. In all breeds studied to date, PRA is recessively inherited.

Affected Curly-Coated Retrievers have been detected at 3-5 years of age and have been seen in the end stage at 6-7 years of age.

References

1.   Rubin LF: Inherited Eye Diseases in Purebred Dogs. Williams & Wilkins, Baltimore, 1989, p 99.

2.   Barnett KC: Comparative aspects of canine hereditary eye disease. Adv Vet Sci Comp Med 20:39, 1976.

3.   ACVO Genetics Committee, 1992 and/or Data from CERF All-Breeds Report, 1991.

DACHSHUND

	DISORDER	INHERITANCE	REFERENCE	BREEDING ADVICE
A.	Dermoid	Not defined	1,7	NO
B.	Endothelial dystrophy	Not defined	2,7	NO
C.	Chronic pigmentary keratitis (pannus)	Autosomal recessive	3,7	NO
D.	Cataract	Not defined	--	NO
E.	Progressive Retinal Atrophy	Not defined	4,7	NO
F.	Multiple ocular defects	Not defined	5-7	NO

Description and Comments

A.   Dermoid

A dermoid is a focal area of normal epidermal tissue that forms in an abnormal location. The lesion generally causes discomfort to the affected animal.

B.   Corneal endothelial dystrophy

An abnormal loss of the inner lining of the cornea that causes progressive fluid retention (edema). With time the edema results in keratitis and decreased vision. This usually does not occur until the animal is older.

C.   Pannus / Chronic superficial keratitis

A bilateral disease of the cornea which usually starts as a grayish haze to the ventral or ventrolateral cornea, followed by the formation of a vascularized subepithelial growth that begins to spread toward the central cornea; pigmentation follows the vascularization. If severe, vision impairment occurs.

D. Cataract

Lens opacity which may affect one or both eyes and may involve the lens partially or completely. In cases where cataracts are complete and affect both eyes, blindness results. The prudent approach is to assume cataracts to be hereditary except in cases known to be associated with trauma, other causes of ocular inflammation, specific metabolic diseases, persistent pupillary membranes, persistent hyaloid or nutritional deficiencies.

E. Progressive Retinal Atrophy (PRA)

A degenerative disease of the retinal visual cells which progresses to blindness. This abnormality may be detected by electroretinogram before it is apparent clinically. In all breeds studied to date, PRA is recessively inherited.

F. Multiple ocular anomalies associated with merling

Microphthalmia is a congenital defect characterized by a small eye with associated defects of the cornea, anterior chamber, lens and/or retina.

Other Conditions Under Consideration

G. Punctate keratitis

Focal circular rings usually affecting the central subepithelial and/or anterior portion of the cornea. There often is an associated dry eye with corneal erosions. The mode of inheritance is unknown.

References

1. Brandsch H, Schmidt V: Analysis of heredity for dermoid in the dog eye. Mh Vet-Med 37:305, 1982.

2. Martin CL, Dice PF: Corneal endothelial dystrophy in the dog. J Am Anim Hosp Assoc 18:327, 1982.

3. Brandsch H, Nicodem K: Heredity of keratitis in long-haired dachshunds. Mh Vet-Med 37:216, 1982.

4. Priester WA: Canine progressive retinal atrophy. Occurrence by age, breed and sex. Am J Vet Res 35:571, 1974.

5.	Dausch O et al: Eye changes in the merle syndrome in the dachshund. Dtsch Tierorxtl Wschr 84:453, 1977.

6.	Sorsby A, Davey JB: Ocular associations of dappling (or merling) in the coat colour of dogs 1. Clinical and genetical data. J Genet 52:425, 1954.

7.	Rubin L: <u>Inherited Eye Diseases in Purebred Dogs</u>. Williams & Wilkins, 1989.

DALMATIAN

	DISORDER	INHERITANCE	REFERENCE	BREEDING ADVICE
A.	Distichiasis	Not defined	1	Breeder option
B.	Entropion	Not defined	1-3	Breeder option
C.	Dermoid	Not defined	2	Breeder option
D.	Glaucoma	Not defined	2,4	No

Description and Comments

A.   Distichiasis

Eyelashes abnormally located in the eyelid margin which may cause ocular irritation. Distichiasis may occur at any time in the life of a dog. It is difficult to make a strong recommendation with regard to breeding dogs with this entity. The hereditary basis has not been established although it seems probable due to the high incidence in some breeds. Reducing the incidence is a logical goal. When diagnosed, distichiasis should be recorded; breeding discretion is advised.

B.   Entropion

A conformational defect resulting in an "in-rolling" of one or more of the eyelids which may cause ocular irritation. It is likely that entropion is influenced by several genes (polygenic), defining the skin and other structures which make up the eyelids, the amount and weight of the skin covering the head and face, the orbital contents, and the conformation of the skull. In the Dalmatian, entropion normally involves the lower lid.

C.   Dermoid

A patch of skin, usually located on the cornea; its presence usually causes ocular irritation and if large can affect vision.

This abnormal development of the cornea has been observed so extensively in some Dalmatian dogs that little corneal tissue remains visible. It has been observed both unilaterally and bilaterally and in more than one dog in a litter on occasion. Surgical correction in most patients helps to return comfort and improve vision.

D.   Glaucoma

Glaucoma is characterized by an elevation of intraocular pressure which, when sustained, causes intraocular damage resulting in blindness. The elevated intraocular pressure occurs because the fluid cannot leave through the iridocorneal angle. Diagnosis and classification of glaucoma requires measurement of the intraocular pressure (tonometry) and examination of the iridocorneal angle (gonioscopy). Neither of these tests are part of a routine breed eye screening exam.

Other Conditions Under Consideration

E.   Pannus / chronic superficial keratitis

A bilateral disease of the cornea which usually starts as a grayish haze to the ventral or ventrolateral cornea, followed by the formation of a vascularized subepithelial growth that begins to spread toward the central cornea; pigmentation follows the vascularization. If severe, vision impairment occurs.

F.   Progressive Retinal Atrophy (PRA)

A degenerative disease of the retinal visual cells which progresses to blindness. This abnormality may be detected by electroretinogram before it is apparent clinically. In all breeds studied to date, PRA is recessively inherited.

G.   Microphthalmia

A developmental anomaly in which the eyeball is abnormally small. This is often associated with other ocular malformations, including defects of the cornea, anterior chamber, lens and/or retina.

H.   Persistent pupillary membranes (PPM)

Persistent blood vessel remnants in the anterior chamber of the eye which fail to regress normally in the neonatal period. These strands may bridge from iris to iris, iris to cornea, iris to lens, or form sheets of tissue in the anterior chamber. The last three forms pose the greatest threat to vision and when severe, vision impairment or blindness may occur.

114

References

1. Rubin LF: <u>Inherited Eye Diseases in Purebred Dogs</u>. Williams & Wilkins, Baltimore, 1989, p107.

2. ACVO Genetics Committee, 1992 and/or Data from CERF All-Breeds Report, 1991.

3. Hodgman SF: Abnormalities and defects in pedigree dogs I. An investigation into the existence of abnormalities in the British Isles. J Small Anim Pract 4:447, 1963.

4. Slater MR, Erb HN: Effects of risk factors and prophylactic treatment on primary glaucoma in the dog. J Am Vet Med Assoc 188:1028, 1986.

DANDIE DINMONT TERRIER

	DISORDER	INHERITANCE	REFERENCE	BREEDING ADVICE
A.	Cataract	Not defined	1	NO
B.	Glaucoma	Not defined	1	NO

Description and Comments

A.   Cataract

Lens opacity which may affect one or both eyes and may involve the lens partially or completely. In cases where cataracts are complete and affect both eyes, blindness results. The prudent approach is to assume cataracts to be hereditary except in cases known to be associated with trauma, other causes of ocular inflammation, specific metabolic diseases, persistent pupillary membranes, persistent hyaloid or nutritional deficiencies.

B.   Glaucoma

Glaucoma is characterized by an elevation of intraocular pressure (IOP) which, when sustained, causes intraocular damage resulting in blindness. The elevated IOP occurs because the fluid cannot leave through the iridocorneal angle. Diagnosis and classification of glaucoma requires measurement of the IOP (tonometry) and examination of the iridocorneal angle (gonioscopy). Neither of these tests are part of a routine breed eye screening exam.

References

There are no references providing detailed descriptions of hereditary ocular conditions of the Dandie Dinmont Terrier breed. The conditions listed above are generally recognized to exist in this breed, as evidenced by repeated references made in general texts.

1.   ACVO Genetics Committee, 1992 and/or Data from CERF All-Breeds Report, 1991.

DOBERMAN PINSCHER

	DISORDER	INHERITANCE	REFERENCE	BREEDING ADVICE
A.	Entropion	Not defined	1	Breeder option
B.	Cataract	Not defined	1	NO
C.	Hyperplastic primary vitreous	Dominant/ incomplete penetrance	1-4	NO
D.	Progressive Retinal Atrophy	Not defined	1	NO
E.	Microphthalmia/ multiple ocular defects	Not defined	1	NO
F.	Eversion of cartilage of third eyelid	Not defined	1	Breeder option

Description and Comments

A. Entropion

A conformational defect resulting in an "in-rolling" of one or more of the eyelids which may cause ocular irritation. It is likely that entropion is influenced by several genes (polygenic), defining the skin and other structures which make up the eyelids, the amount and weight of the skin covering the head and face, the orbital contents, and the conformation of the skull.

Entropion in the Doberman Pinscher can be unilateral or bilateral and usually occurs within the first year of age.

B.   Cataract

Lens opacity which may affect one or both eyes and may involve the lens partially or completely. In cases where cataracts are complete and affect both eyes, blindness results. The prudent approach is to assume cataracts to be hereditary except in cases known to be associated with trauma, other causes of ocular inflammation, specific metabolic diseases, persistent pupillary membranes, persistent hyaloid or nutritional deficiencies.

Cataracts have been infrequently observed in the Doberman Pinscher and there is no specific location attributed to cataracts within the Doberman lens. Most cataracts are bilateral, usually observed within the first two years of life, and may cause significant vision loss.

C.   Persistent hyperplastic primary vitreous (PHPV)

A congenital defect resulting from abnormalities in the development and regression of the hyaloid artery (the primary vitreous) and the interaction of this blood vessel with the posterior lens capsule/cortex during embryogenesis.

PHPV has been extensively studied in the Doberman Pinscher in Europe. This disorder has been observed occasionally in the Doberman Pinscher in the United States.

D.   Progressive Retinal Atrophy (PRA)

A degenerative disease of the retinal visual cells which progresses to blindness. This abnormality may be detected by electroretinogram before it is apparent clinically. In all breeds studied to date, PRA is recessively inherited.

E.   Microphthalmia

A developmental anomaly in which the eyeball is abnormally small. This is often associated with other ocular malformations, including defects of the cornea, anterior chamber, lens and/or retina.

F.   Eversion of the cartilage of the third eyelid

A scroll-like curling of the cartilage of the third eyelid, usually everting the margin. The condition may occur in one or both eyes and may cause mild ocular irritation.

References

1. ACVO Genetics Committee, 1992 and/or data from CERF All-Breeds Report, 1991.

2. Stades FC: Persistent hyperplastic tunica vasculosa lentis and persistent hyperplastic primary vitreous (PHTVL/PHPV) in ninety closely related Pinschers. J Am Anim Hosp Assoc 16:739, 1980.

3. Stades FC: Persistent hyperplastic tunica vasculosa lentis and persistent hyperplastic primary vitreous in Doberman Pinschers: Genetic aspects. J Am Anim Hosp Assoc 19:957, 1983.

4. Peiffer RL, Gelatt KN, Gwin RM: Persistent primary vitreous and a pigmented cataract in a dog. J Am Anim Hosp Assoc 13:478, 1977.

5. Bergsjo T et al: Congenital blindness with developmental anomalies, including retinal dysplasia, in Doberman Pinscher dogs. J Am Vet Med Assoc 184:1383, 1984.

6. Arnvjerg J and Jensen OA: Spontaneous microphthalmia in two Doberman puppies with anterior chamber cleavage syndrome. J Am Anim Hosp Assoc 18:481, 1982.

ENGLISH COCKER SPANIEL

	DISORDER	INHERITANCE	REFERENCE	BREEDING ADVICE
A.	Ectropion	Not defined	--	Breeder option
B.	Distichiasis	Not defined	--	Breeder option
C.	Imperforate lacrimal punctum	Not defined	--	Breeder option
D.	Persistent pupillary membrane	Not defined	--	Breeder option
E.	Cataract	Not defined	1	NO
F.	Progressive Retinal Atrophy	Autosomal recessive	2	NO
G.	Retinal dysplasia - folds	Not defined	3	Breeder option

Description and Comments

A.   Ectropion

A conformational defect resulting in eversion of the eyelids which may cause ocular irritation. It is likely that ectropion is influenced by several genes (polygenic) defining the skin and other structures which make up the eyelids, the amount and weight of the skin covering the head and face, the orbital contents and the conformation of the skull.

B.   Distichiasis

Eyelashes abnormally located in the eyelid margin which may cause ocular irritation. Distichiasis may occur at any time in the life of a dog. It is difficult to make a strong recommendation with regard to breeding dogs with this entity. The hereditary basis has not been established, although it seems probable due to the high incidence in some breeds. Reducing the incidence is a logical goal. When diagnosed, distichiasis should be recorded; breeding discretion is advised.

C.   Imperforate lacrimal punctum

A developmental abnormality resulting in failure of opening of the lacrimal duct adjacent to the eye. The lower duct is more frequently affected. This defect usually results in epiphora, a spillover of tears onto the face.

D.   Persistent pupillary membrane (PPM)

Persistent blood vessel remnants in the anterior chamber of the eye which fail to regress normally in the neonatal period. These strands may bridge from iris to iris, iris to cornea, iris to lens, or form sheets of tissue in the anterior chamber. The last three forms pose the greatest threat to vision and when severe, vision impairment or blindness may occur.

E.   Cataract

Lens opacity which may affect one or both eyes and may involve the lens partially or completely. In cases where cataracts are complete and affect both eyes, blindness results. The prudent approach is to assume cataracts to be hereditary except in cases known to be associated with trauma, other causes of ocular inflammation, specific metabolic diseases, persistent pupillary membranes, persistent hyaloid or nutritional deficiencies.

Congenital cataracts have been reported in red cocker spaniels, presumably English cocker spaniels, in Denmark. The cataracts affected the anterior capsule; in some cases the cortex and/or nucleus were opaque. Associated findings in some dogs were persistent pupillary membrane (PPM) and/or microphthalmia. It is likely that these cataracts are part of a syndrome characterized by multiple congenital ocular anomalies. The condition is familial, but a specific mode of inheritance has not been defined.

F.   Progressive Retinal Atrophy (PRA)

A degenerative disease of the retinal visual cells which progresses to blindness. This abnormality may be detected by electroretinogram before it is apparent clinically. In all breeds studied to date, PRA is recessively inherited.

This photoreceptor degeneration is characterized by slow death of visual cells following their normal development. Early fundus abnormalities usually appear after 4 years of age. The ERG (electroretinogram) shows marked functional abnormalities indicative of a progressive rod-cone degeneration. The age for early diagnosis by ERG is after 18 months of age.

Studies have shown that PRA in the English cocker spaniel is inherited as autosomal recessive. The mutation is allelic to that present in miniature poodles and American cocker spaniels and the locus is termed the progressive rod-cone degeneration (*prcd*) gene.

G.   Retinal dysplasia - folds

Abnormal development of the retina present at birth and recognized to have three forms:

1) Retinal dysplasia - **folds**: linear, triangular, curved or curvilinear foci of retinal folding that may be single or multiple.
2) Retinal dysplasia - **geographic**: any irregularly shaped area of abnormal retinal development, representing changes not accountable by simple folding.
3) Retinal dysplasia - **detachment**: either of the above described forms of retinal dysplasia associated with separation (detachment) of the retina.

The two latter forms are associated with vision impairment or blindness. Retinal dysplasia is known to be inherited in many breeds. The genetic relationship between the three forms of the disease is not known for all breeds.

Other Conditions Under Consideration

H.   Glaucoma

Glaucoma is characterized by an elevation of intraocular pressure (IOP) which, when sustained, causes intraocular damage resulting in blindness. The elevated IOP occurs because the fluid cannot leave through the iridocorneal angle. Diagnosis and classification of glaucoma requires measurement of the intraocular pressure (tonometry) and examination of the iridocorneal angle (gonioscopy). Neither of these tests are part of a routine breed eye screening exam.

Glaucoma in the English cocker spaniel is recognized in England. The frequency and significance of this disease in the breed in the United States is not known, but is probably low.

References

1.   Oleson HP et al: Congenital hereditary cataract in cocker spaniels. J Sm Anim Pract 15:741, 1974.

2.   Aguirre GD, Acland GM: Variation in retinal degeneration phenotype inherited at the *prcd* locus. Exp Eye Res 46:663, 1988.

3.   ACVO Genetics Committee, 1992 and/or Data from CERF All-Breeds Report, 1991.

4.   Bedford PGC: A gonioscopic study of the iridocorneal angle in the English and American breeds of Cocker spaniel and the Basset Hound. J Sm Anim Pract 18:631, 1977.

ENGLISH SETTER

	DISORDER	INHERITANCE	REFERENCE	BREEDING ADVICE
A.	Ectropion	Not defined	1	Breeder option
B.	Macroblepharon	Not defined	1	NO
C.	Progressive Retinal Atrophy	Not defined	1	NO

Description and Comments

A.   Ectropion

A conformational defect resulting in eversion of the eyelids, which may cause ocular irritation due to exposure. It is likely that ectropion is influenced by several genes (polygenic) defining the skin and other structures which make up the eyelids, the amount and weight of the skin covering the head and face, the orbital contents and the conformation of the skull.

B.   Macroblepharon

Abnormally large eyelid opening; may lead to secondary conditions associated with corneal exposure.

C.   Progressive Retinal Atrophy (PRA)

A degenerative disease of the retinal visual cells which progresses to blindness. This abnormality may be detected by electroretinogram before it is apparent clinically. In all breeds studied to date, PRA is recessively inherited.

References

There are no references providing detailed descriptions of hereditary ocular conditions of the English Setter breed. The conditions listed above are generally recognized to exist in this breed, as evidenced by repeated references made in general texts.

1.   ACVO Genetics Committee, 1992 and/or Data from CERF All-Breeds Report, 1991.

ENGLISH SPRINGER SPANIEL

	DISORDER	INHERITANCE	REFERENCE	BREEDING ADVICE
A.	Entropion	Not defined	1	Breeder option
B.	Cataract	Not defined	1,2	NO
C.	Retinal dysplasia - folds - geographic - detachment	Autosomal recessive	3,4	NO
D.	Progressive Retinal Atrophy	Not defined	5	NO

Description and Comments

A.   Entropion

A conformational defect resulting in an "in-rolling" of one or more of the eyelids which may cause ocular irritation. It is likely that entropion is influenced by several genes (polygenic), defining the skin and other structures which make up the eyelids, the amount and weight of the skin covering the head and face, the orbital contents, and the conformation of the skull. In the Springer Spaniel this usually involves the lower lateral lid margin.

B.   Cataract

Lens opacity which may affect one or both eyes and may involve the lens partially or completely. In cases where cataracts are complete and affect both eyes, blindness results. The prudent approach is to assume cataracts to be hereditary except in cases known to be associated with trauma, other causes of ocular inflammation, specific metabolic diseases, persistent pupillary membranes, persistent hyaloid or nutritional deficiencies. Cataract in the English Springer Spaniel is reported to be a familial trait usually involving the posterior subcapsular region of the lens that progresses slowly.

125

C. Retinal Dysplasia

Abnormal development of the retina present at birth and recognized to have three forms:

　　1) Retinal dysplasia - **folds**: linear, triangular, curved or curvilinear foci of retinal folding that may be single or multiple.
　　2)Retinal dysplasia - **geographic**: any irregularly shaped area of abnormal retinal development, representing changes not accountable by simple folding.
　　3) Retinal dysplasia - **detachment**: either of the above described forms of retinal dysplasia associated with separation (detachment) of the retina.

The two latter forms are associated with vision impairment or blindness. Retinal dysplasia is known to be inherited in many breeds. The genetic relationship between the three forms of the disease is not known for all breeds.

D. Progressive Retinal Atrophy (PRA)

A degenerative disease of the retinal visual cells which progresses to blindness. This abnormality may be detected by electroretinogram before it is apparent clinically. In all breeds studied to date, PRA is recessively inherited.

PRA in the English Springer Spaniel appears to be similar to that seen in the English Cocker Spaniel, with onset of clinical signs at 3 to 5 years of age.

References

1.　ACVO Genetics Committee, 1992 and/or Data from CERF All-Breeds Report, 1991.

2.　Rubin LF: Inherited Eye Diseases in Purebred Dogs. Williams and Wilkins, Baltimore, 1989, p124.

3.　Schmidt GM et al: Inheritance of retinal dysplasia in the English Springer spaniel. J Am Vet Med Assoc 174:1089, 1979.

4.　Lavach JD et al: Retinal dysplasia in the English Springer spaniel. J Am Anim Hosp Assoc 14:192, 1978.

5.　Barnett KC: Canine retinopathies III. The other breeds. J Sm Anim Pract 6:185, 1965.

ENGLISH TOY SPANIEL
(King Charles, Prince Charles, Ruby, Blenheim)

	DISORDER	INHERITANCE	REFERENCE	BREEDING ADVICE
A.	Entropion	Not defined	1	Breeder option
B.	Corneal dystrophy	Not defined	1	Breeder option
C.	Cataract	Not defined	1,2	NO
D.	Retinal dysplasia - folds	Not defined	1	Breeder option

Description and Comments

A. Entropion

A conformational defect resulting in "in-rolling" of one or more of the eyelids which may cause ocular irritation. It is likely that entropion is influenced by several genes (polygenic), defining the skin and other structures which make up the eyelids, the amount and weight of the skin covering the head and face, the orbital contents and the conformation of the skull.

B. Corneal dystrophy

A non-inflammatory corneal opacity (white to gray) present in one or more of the corneal layers; usually inherited and bilateral. In these dogs, lesions are circular or semicircular central crystalline deposits in the anterior corneal stroma that appear between 2 and 5 years of age. It may be associated with exophthalmos and lagophthalmos common in these dogs.

C. Cataract

Lens opacity which may affect one or both eyes and may involve the lens partially or completely. In cases where cataracts are complete and affect both eyes, blindness results. The prudent approach is to assume cataracts to be hereditary except in cases known to be associated with trauma, other causes of ocular inflammation, specific metabolic diseases, persistent pupillary membrane, persistent hyaloid or nutritional deficiencies. Onset is at an early age (less than 6 months), affecting the cortex and nucleus; progresses rapidly to complete cataract, resulting in blindness.

D.   Retinal Dysplasia

Abnormal development of the retina present at birth and recognized to have three forms:

> 1) Retinal dysplasia - **folds**: linear, triangular, curved or curvilinear foci of retinal folding that may be single or multiple.
> 2) Retinal dysplasia - **geographic**: any irregularly shaped area of abnormal retinal development, representing changes not accountable by simple folding.
> 3) Retinal dysplasia - **detachment**: either of the above described forms of retinal dysplasia associated with separation (detachment) of the retina.

The two latter forms are associated with vision impairment or blindness. Retinal dysplasia is known to be inherited in many breeds. The genetic relationship between the three forms of the disease is not known for all breeds.

References

There are no references providing detailed descriptions of hereditary ocular conditions of the English Toy Spaniel breed. The conditions listed above are generally recognized to exist in the breed, as evidenced by repeated references made in general texts.

1.   ACVO Genetics Committee, 1992 and/or Data from CERF All-Breeds Report, 1991.

2.   Rubin LF: Inherited Eye Diseases in Purebred Dogs. Williams and Wilkins, Baltimore, 1989.

FIELD SPANIEL

	DISORDER	INHERITANCE	REFERENCE	BREEDING ADVICE
A.	Cataract	Not defined	1	NO
B.	Progressive Retinal Atrophy	Not defined	1	NO
C.	Retinal dysplasia - folds - geographic	Not defined	1	Breeder option

Description and Comments

A.   Cataract

Lens opacity which may affect one or both eyes and may involve the lens partially or completely. In cases where cataracts are complete and affect both eyes, blindness results. The prudent approach is to assume cataracts to be hereditary except in cases known to be associated with trauma, other causes of ocular inflammation, specific metabolic diseases, persistent pupillary membrane, persistent hyaloid or nutritional deficiencies. Multiple focal cortical cataracts have been seen in 3 year old dogs. These rarely progress to total cataract.

B.   Progressive Retinal Atrophy (PRA)

A degenerative disease of the retinal visual cells which progresses to blindness. This abnormality may be detected by electroretinogram before it is apparent clinically. In all breeds studied to date, PRA is recessively inherited. In the Field Spaniel, the disease may become clinically apparent in 5 year old dogs. A band of normal retina dorsal to the optic disc may persist late into the disease, preserving some vision.

C.   Retinal Dysplasia

Abnormal development of the retina present at birth and recognized to have three forms:

1) Retinal dysplasia - **folds**: linear, triangular, curved or curvilinear foci of retinal folding that may be single or multiple.

2) Retinal dysplasia - **geographic**: any irregularly shaped area of abnormal retinal development, representing changes not accountable by simple folding.

3) Retinal dysplasia - **detachment**: either of the above described forms of retinal dysplasia associated with separation (detachment) of the retina.

The two latter forms are associated with vision impairment or blindness. Retinal dysplasia is known to be inherited in many breeds. The genetic relationship between the three forms of the disease is not known for all breeds.

Two types of retinal dysplasia have been described in the Field Spaniel, multifocal and geographic. The multifocal folds resemble those seen in the Cocker Spaniel. Geographic lesions resemble the larger dysplastic areas such as seen in the English Springer Spaniel and are associated with vitreous liquefaction.

References

There are no references providing detailed descriptions of hereditary ocular conditions of the Field Spaniel breed. The conditions listed above are generally recognized to exist in this breed, as evidenced by repeated references made in general texts.

1.   ACVO Genetics Committee, 1992 and/or Data from CERF All-Breeds Report, 1991.

FLAT-COATED RETRIEVER

	DISORDER	INHERITANCE	REFERENCE	BREEDING ADVICE
A.	Entropion	Not defined	--	Breeder option
B.	Distichiasis	Not defined	1	Breeder option
C.	Cataract	Not defined	--	NO
D.	Progressive Retinal Atrophy	Not defined	--	NO

Description and Comments

A.   Entropion

A conformational defect resulting in an "in-rolling" of one or more of the eyelids which may cause ocular irritation. It is likely that entropion is influenced by several genes (polygenic), defining the skin and other structures which make up the eyelids, the amount and weight of the skin covering the head and face, the orbital contents, and the conformation of the skull. Selection should be directed against entropion and toward head conformation that minimizes or eliminates the likelihood of the defect.

B.   Distichiasis

Eyelashes abnormally located in the eyelid margin which may cause ocular irritation. Distichiasis may occur at any time in the life of a dog. It is difficult to make a strong recommendation with regard to breeding dogs with this entity. The hereditary basis has not been established, although it seems probable due to the high incidence in some breeds. Reducing the incidence is a logical goal. When diagnosed, distichiasis should be recorded; breeding discretion is advised.

C.   Cataract

Lens opacity which may affect one or both eyes and may involve the lens partially or completely. In cases where cataracts are complete and affect both eyes, blindness results. The prudent approach is to assume cataracts to be hereditary except in cases

131

known to be associated with trauma, other causes of ocular inflammation, specific metabolic diseases, persistent pupillary membranes, persistent hyaloid or nutritional deficiencies. The exact frequency and significance of cataracts in the breed is not known, although it is probably low.

D.   Progressive Retinal Atrophy (PRA)

A degenerative disease of the retinal visual cells which progresses to blindness. This abnormality may be detected by electroretinogram before it is apparent clinically. In all breeds studied to date, PRA is recessively inherited. The exact frequency and significance of PRA in the breed is not known, although it is probably low.

References

There are no references providing detailed descriptions of hereditary ocular conditions of the Flat-Coated Retriever breed. The conditions listed above are generally recognized to exist in this breed, as evidenced by repeated references made in general texts.

1.   ACVO Genetics Committee, 1992 and/or Data from CERF All-Breeds Report, 1991.

FOX TERRIER

	DISORDER	INHERITANCE	REFERENCE	BREEDING ADVICE
A.	Glaucoma	Not defined	1	NO
B.	Cataract	Not defined	2	NO
C.	Lens luxation	Not defined	3-5	NO

Description and Comments

A. Glaucoma

Glaucoma is characterized by an elevation of intraocular pressure (IOP) which, when sustained, causes intraocular damage resulting in blindness. The elevated IOP occurs because the fluid cannot leave through the iridocorneal angle. Diagnosis and classification of glaucoma requires measurement of the intraocular pressure (tonometry) and examination of the iridocorneal angle (gonioscopy). Neither of these tests are part of a routine breed eye screening exam.

B. Cataract

Lens opacity which may affect one or both eyes and may involve the lens partially or completely. In cases where cataracts are complete and affect both eyes, blindness results. The prudent approach is to assume cataracts to be hereditary except in cases known to be associated with trauma, other causes of ocular inflammation, specific metabolic diseases, persistent pupillary membranes, persistent hyaloid or nutritional deficiencies. The cataracts observed in this breed begin in the posterior subcapsular region and are progressive.

C. Lens luxation

Partial (subluxation) or complete displacement of the lens from the normal anatomic site behind the pupil. Lens luxation not associated with trauma or inflammation is presumed to be inherited. Lens luxation may result in elevated intraocular pressure (glaucoma) causing vision impairment or blindness.

References

1. Martin CL, Wyman M: Primary glaucoma in the dog. Vet Clin North Amer 8:257, 1978.

2. ACVO Genetics Committee, 1992 and/or Data from CERF All-Breeds Report, 1991.

3. Formston C: Observations on subluxation and luxation of the crystalline lens in the dog. J Comp Pathol 55:168, 1945.

4. Lawson: Luxation of the crystalline lens in the dog. J Sm Anim Pract 10:461, 1969.

5. Curtis, Barnett: Primary lens luxation in the dog. J Sm Anim Pract 21:657, 1980.

FRENCH BULLDOG

	DISORDER	INHERITANCE	REFERENCE	BREEDING ADVICE
A.	Distichiasis	Not defined	1,3	Breeder option
B.	Entropion	Not defined	1,2	Breeder option
C.	Cataract	Not defined	1,3	NO

Description and Comments

A. Distichiasis

Eyelashes abnormally located in the eyelid margin which may cause ocular irritation. Distichiasis may occur at any time in the life of a dog. It is difficult to make a strong recommendation with regard to breeding dogs with this entity. The hereditary basis has not been established although it seems probable due to the high incidence in some breeds. Reducing the incidence is a logical goal. When diagnosed, distichiasis should be recorded; breeding discretion is advised.

B. Entropion

A conformational defect resulting in an "in-rolling" of one or more of the eyelids which may cause ocular irritation. It is likely that entropion is influenced by several genes (polygenic), defining the skin and other structures which make up the eyelids, the amount and weight of the skin covering the head and face, the orbital contents, and the conformation of the skull.

In the French Bulldog, entropion normally involves the lower eyelid and has been observed in the nasal half (medial canthus region).

C. Cataract

Lens opacity which may affect one or both eyes and may involve the lens partially or completely. In cases where cataracts are complete and affect both eyes, blindness results. The prudent approach is to assume cataracts to be hereditary except in cases known to be associated with trauma, other causes of ocular inflammation, specific metabolic diseases, persistent pupillary membranes, persistent hyaloid or nutritional deficiencies.

In the French Bulldog, this opacity has been observed originating in the equatorial and/or posterior cortical regions. The cataract formation is usually bilateral, occurs in young dogs (6 months to 2 years), and rapidly progresses to completion. Posterior lenticonus has also been observed.

References

1. Rubin LE: <u>Inherited Eye Diseases in Purebred Dogs</u>. Williams and Wilkins, Baltimore, 1989, p137.

2. Johnston DE, Cox B: The incidence in purebred dogs in Australia of abnormalities that may be inherited. Aust Vet J 46:465, 1970.

3. ACVO Genetics Committee, 1992 and/or Data from CERF All-Breeds Report, 1991.

GERMAN SHEPHERD

	DISORDER	INHERITANCE	REFERENCE	BREEDING ADVICE
A.	Eversion of cartilage of third eyelid	Not defined	1,2	Breeder option
B.	Pannus	Not defined	3-6	Breeder option
C.	Cataract			
	1. Congenital	Autosomal dominant	7	NO
	2. Cortical	Autosomal recessive	8	NO
D.	Progressive Retinal Atrophy	Not defined	8-11	NO
E.	Optic nerve hypoplasia / Micropapilla	Not defined	1,2	NO
F.	Retinal dysplasia - folds - geographic	Not defined	1	NO

Description and Comments

A.   Eversion of the cartilage of the third eyelid

A scroll-like curling of the cartilage of the third eyelid, usually everting the margin. This condition may occur in one or both eyes and may cause mild ocular irritation.

B.   Pannus / Chronic superficial keratitis

A bilateral disease of the cornea which usually starts as a grayish haze to the ventral or ventrolateral cornea, followed by the formation of a vascularized subepithelial growth that begins to spread toward the central cornea; pigmentation follows the vascularization. If severe, vision impairment occurs.

The German Shepherd dog has a higher incidence of pannus than any other breed. While environment may play a contributing role, an inherited predisposition must be considered.

C.   Cataract

Lens opacity which may affect one or both eyes and may involve the lens partially or completely. In cases where cataracts are complete and affect both eyes, blindness results. The prudent approach is to assume cataracts to be hereditary except in cases known to be associated with trauma, other causes of ocular inflammation, specific metabolic diseases, persistent pupillary membranes, persistent hyaloid or nutritional deficiencies.

1. Congenital: Reported by von Hippel in Germany in 1930, these cataracts are present at birth and visible when the eyes open. They are usually non-progressive. Test breedings indicate an autosomal dominant mode of transmission. The occurrence is rare.

2. Cortical: Reported by Barnett in Great Britain, opacities are first apparent at 8-12 weeks of age, in the posterior cortex and progress to involve the Y-sutures and nucleus. The equatorial subcapsular cortex is unaffected. No progression is noted after 1-2 years of age. Test breeding suggests an autosomal recessive mode of inheritance.

D.   Progressive Retinal Atrophy (PRA)

A degenerative disease of the retinal visual cells which progresses to blindness. This abnormality may be detected by electroretinogram before it is apparent clinically. In all breeds studied to date, PRA is recessively inherited.

E.   Optic nerve hypoplasia

A congenital defect of the optic nerve which causes blindness and abnormal pupil response in the affected eye. May be unable to differentiate from micropapilla on a routine (dilated) screening ophthalmoscopic exam.

F.   Retinal Dysplasia

Abnormal development of the retina present at birth and recognized to have three forms:

1) Retinal dysplasia - **folds**: linear, triangular, curved or curvilinear foci of retinal folding that may be single or multiple.
2) Retinal dysplasia - **geographic**: any irregularly shaped area of abnormal retinal development, representing changes not accountable by simple folding.
3) Retinal dysplasia - **detachment**: either of the above described forms of retinal dysplasia associated with separation (detachment) of the retina.

The two latter forms are associated with vision impairment or blindness. Retinal dysplasia is known to be inherited in many breeds. The genetic relationship between the three forms of the disease is not known for all breeds.

Other Conditions Under Consideration

G.   Corneal dystrophy

A non-inflammatory corneal opacity (white to gray) present in one or more of the corneal layers; usually inherited and bilateral.

H.   Dermoid

A patch of skin, usually located on the cornea; its presence usually causes ocular irritation.

References

1.   ACVO Genetics Committee, 1992 and/or Data from CERF All-Breeds Report, 1991.

2.   Rubin LF: Inherited Eye Diseases in Purebred Dogs. Williams and Wilkins, Baltimore, 1989, p138.

3.   Campbell LH et al: Chronic superficial keratitis in dogs: Detection of cellular hypersensitivity. Am J Vet Res 36:669, 1975.

4.   Eichenbaum JD et al: Immunohistochemical staining patterns of canine eyes affected with chronic superficial keratitis. Am J Vet Res 47:1952, 1986.

5. Slatter DH et al: Uberreiter's syndrome (chronic superficial keratitis) in dogs in the Rocky Mountain area: a study of 463 cases. J Small Anim Pract 18:757, 1977.

6. Uberreiter O: (A particular form of keratitis [chronic superficial keratitis] in dogs). Wien Tierarztl Mschr 48:65, 1961.

7. von Hippel E: (Embryological investigation of hereditary congenital cataract, of lamellar cataract in dogs as well as a peculiar form of capsular cataract). Graefes Arch Ophthalmol 124:300, 1930.

8. Barnett KC: Hereditary cataract in the German shepherd dog. J Sm Anim Pract 27:387, 1986.

9. Barnett KC: Canine retinopathies III. The other breeds. J Sm Anim Pract 6:185, 1965.

10. Hodgman SFJ: Abnormalities and defects in pedigree dogs I. An investigation into the existence of abnormalities in pedigree dogs in the British Isles. J Sm Anim Pract 4:447, 1963.

11. Priester WA: Canine progressive retinal atrophy. Occurrence by age, breed and sex. Am J Vet Res 35:571, 1974.

GERMAN SHORTHAIRED POINTER

	DISORDER	INHERITANCE	REFERENCE	BREEDING ADVICE
A.	Entropion	Not defined	1	Breeder option
B.	Eversion of cartilage of third eyelid	Not defined	2	Breeder option
C.	Cataract	Not defined	1	NO
D.	Progressive Retinal Atrophy	Not defined	3	NO

Description and Comments

A. Entropion

A conformational defect resulting in an "in-rolling" of one or more of the eyelids which may cause ocular irritation. It is likely that entropion is influenced by several genes (polygenic), defining the skin and other structures which make up the eyelids, the amount and weight of the skin covering the head and face, the orbital contents, and the conformation of the skull.

B. Eversion of the cartilage of the third eyelid

A scroll-like curling of the cartilage of the third eyelid, usually everting the margin. This condition may occur in one or both eyes and may cause mild ocular irritation.

C. Cataract

Lens opacity which may affect one or both eyes and may involve the lens partially or completely. In cases where cataracts are complete and affect both eyes, blindness results. The prudent approach is to assume cataracts to be hereditary except in cases known to be associated with trauma, other causes of ocular inflammation, specific metabolic diseases, persistent pupillary membranes, persistent hyaloid or nutritional deficiencies.

D.   Progressive Retinal Atrophy (PRA)

A degenerative disease of the retinal visual cells which progresses to blindness. This abnormality may be detected by electroretinogram before it is apparent clinically. In all breeds studied to date, PRA is recessively inherited.

References

1.   ACVO Genetics Committee, 1992 and/or Data from CERF All-Breeds Report, 1991.

2.   Martin CL, Leach R: Everted membrane nictitans in German shorthaired pointers. J Am Vet Med Assoc 157:1229, 1970.

3.   Priester WA: Canine progressive retinal atrophy: Occurrence by age, breed and sex. Am J Vet Res 35:571, 1974.

GERMAN WIREHAIRED POINTER

	DISORDER	INHERITANCE	REFERENCE	BREEDING ADVICE
A.	Entropion	Not defined	1	Breeder option

Description and Comments

A.   Entropion

A conformational defect resulting in an "in-rolling" of one or more of the eyelids which may cause ocular irritation. It is likely that entropion is influenced by several genes (polygenic), defining the skin and other structures which make up the eyelids, the amount and weight of the skin covering the head and face, the orbital contents, and the conformation of the skull.

References

There are no references providing detailed descriptions of hereditary ocular conditions of the German Wirehaired Pointer breed. The conditions listed above are generally recognized to exist in this breed, as evidenced by repeated references made in general texts.

1.   ACVO Genetics Committee, 1992 and/or Data from CERF All-Breeds Report, 1991.

GIANT SCHNAUZER

	DISORDER	INHERITANCE	REFERENCE	BREEDING ADVICE
A.	Cataract	Not defined	--	NO
B.	Progressive Retinal Atrophy	Not defined	--	NO
C.	Retinal dysplasia - folds	Not defined	--	Breeder option

Description and Comments

A.   Cataract

Lens opacity which may affect one or both eyes and may involve the lens partially or completely. In cases where cataracts are complete and affect both eyes, blindness results. The prudent approach is to assume cataracts to be hereditary except in cases known to be associated with trauma, other causes of ocular inflammation, specific metabolic diseases, persistent pupillary membranes, persistent hyaloid or nutritional deficiencies.

B.   Progressive Retinal Atrophy (PRA)

A degenerative disease of the retinal visual cells which progresses to blindness. This abnormality may be detected by electroretinogram before it is apparent clinically. In all breeds studied to date, PRA is recessively inherited.

C.   Retinal dysplasia

Abnormal development of the retina present at birth and recognized to have three forms:

1) Retinal dysplasia - **folds**: linear, triangular, curved or curvilinear foci of retinal folding that may be single or multiple.
2) Retinal dysplasia - **geographic**: any irregularly shaped area of abnormal retinal development, representing changes not accountable by simple folding.
3) Retinal dysplasia - **detachment**: either of the above described forms of

retinal dysplasia associated with separation (detachment) of the retina.

The two latter forms are associated with vision impairment or blindness. Retinal dysplasia is known to be inherited in many breeds. The genetic relationship between the three forms of the disease is not known for all breeds.

Other Conditions Under Consideration

D.   Goniodysgenesis

A congenital anomaly characterized by the persistence of a sheet of tissue between the base of the iris and the inner corneoscleral junction in the area where drainage normally occurs.

E.   Persistent hyperplastic primary vitreous (PHPV)

A congenital defect resulting from abnormalities in the development and regression of the hyaloid artery (the primary vitreous) and the interaction of this blood vessel with the posterior lens capsule/cortex during embryogenesis. This condition is often associated with **persistent tunica vasculosa lentis (PTVL)** which results from failure of regression of the embryologic vascular network which surrounds the developing lens.

F.   Vitreal degeneration

A liquefaction of the vitreous gel which may predispose to retinal detachment.

References

There are no references providing detailed descriptions of hereditary ocular conditions of the Giant Schnauzer breed. The conditions listed above are generally recognized to exist in this breed, as evidenced by repeated references made in general texts.

1.   ACVO Genetics Committee, 1992 and/or Data from CERF All-Breeds Report, 1991.

GOLDEN RETRIEVER

	DISORDER	INHERITANCE	REFERENCE	BREEDING ADVICE
A.	Entropion	Not defined	1	Breeder option
B.	Distichiasis	Not defined	1	Breeder option
C.	Cataract	Not defined	1,5,6,7	NO
D.	Progressive Retinal Atrophy	Autosomal recessive	1,2,3	NO
E.	Central Progressive Retinal Atrophy	Not defined	4	NO

Description and Comments

A.   Entropion

A conformational defect resulting in an "in-rolling" of one or more of the eyelids which may cause ocular irritation. It is likely that entropion is influenced by several genes (polygenic), defining the skin and other structures which make up the eyelids, the amount and weight of the skin covering the head and face, the orbital contents, and the conformation of the skull.

Entropion in the Golden retriever usually involves the lower eyelids and has been increasingly observed with concurrent enophthalmos. Surgical correction is required in this breed to remove the discomfort.

B.   Distichiasis

Eyelashes abnormally located in the eyelid margin which may cause ocular irritation. Distichiasis may occur at any time in the life of a dog. It is difficult to make a strong recommendation with regard to breeding dogs with this entity. The hereditary basis has not been established although it seems probable due to the high incidence in some breeds. Reducing the incidence is a logical goal. When diagnosed, distichiasis should be recorded; breeding discretion is advised.

C.   Cataract

Lens opacity which may affect one or both eyes and may involve the lens partially or completely. In cases where cataracts are complete and affect both eyes, blindness results. The prudent approach is to assume cataracts to be hereditary except in cases known to be associated with trauma, other causes of ocular inflammation, specific metabolic diseases, persistent pupillary membranes, persistent hyaloid or nutritional deficiencies.

The most common cataract reported in the Golden Retriever is a posterior polar (posterior cortical) cataract. These are generally bilateral, although an occasional unilateral affliction may be observed. These focal opacities will occasionally remain stationary. These cataracts are usually observed between 9 months and 3 years of age. A more generalized cataract is also observed in this breed and is not always associated with the previously mentioned polar cataract. There are also cataract changes involving the Y sutures which may or may not progress.

The existence of cataracts in the Golden retriever, often with limited clinical significance, presents problems with breeder recognition as the majority of these dogs do not evidence visual impairment. It is strongly recommended that all Golden retrievers that are used in breeding programs be examined annually as cataract changes have been observed in multiple locations of the lens and variable age of onset.

D.   Progressive Retinal Atrophy (PRA)

A degenerative disease of the retinal visual cells which progresses to blindness. This abnormality may be detected by electroretinogram before it is apparent clinically. In all breeds studied to date, PRA is recessively inherited.

E.   Central Progressive Retinal Atrophy (CPRA)

A progressive retinal degeneration in which photoreceptor death occurs secondary to disease of the underlying pigment epithelium. Progression is slow and some animals never lose vision. CPRA occurs in England, but is uncommon elsewhere.

Other Conditions Under Consideration

F.   Retinal dysplasia

Abnormal development of the retina present at birth and recognized to have three forms:

1) Retinal dysplasia - **folds**: linear, triangular, curved or curvilinear foci of retinal folding that may be single or multiple.

2) Retinal dysplasia - **geographic**: any irregularly shaped area of abnormal retinal development representing changes not accountable by simple folding.

3) Retinal dysplasia - **detachment**: either of the above described forms of retinal dysplasia associated with separation (detachment) of the retina.

The two latter forms are associated with vision impairment or blindness. Retinal dysplasia is known to be inherited in many breeds. The genetic relationship between the three forms of the disease is not known for all breeds.

The fold form has been observed in the Golden retriever.

G.   Pigmentary uveitis

A unique uveitis observed in the Golden retriever, unassociated with other ocular or systemic disorders. Adhesions develop between iris and lens and the peripheral iris and cornea. Other complications include secondary cataract and obstructive glaucoma. Pigment dispersion (exfoliation) occurs across the anterior lens capsule from the pigmented cells of the posterior iris.

H.   Glaucoma

Glaucoma is characterized by an elevation of intraocular pressure (IOP) which, when sustained, causes intraocular damage resulting in blindness. The elevated intraocular pressure occurs because the fluid cannot leave through the iridocorneal angle. Diagnosis and classification of glaucoma requires measurement of the IOP (tonometry) and examination of the iridocorneal angle (gonioscopy). Neither of these tests are part of a routine breed eye screening exam.

I.   Iris cysts

Fluid filled sacs arising from the posterior surface of the iris, to which they may remain attached or break free and float into the anterior chamber. Usually occur in mature dogs.

This disorder may be observed in any breed but retriever breeds tend to be predisposed. There is usually no effect on vision unless the cysts are heavily clustered and impinge on the pupillary area. Less frequently, the cysts may rupture and adhere to the cornea or anterior lens capsule.

References

1.   ACVO Genetics Committee, 1992 and/or Data from CERF All-Breeds Report, 1991.

2.   Gelatt KN: Description and diagnosis of progressive retinal atrophy. Norden News 24, 1974.

3.   Barnett KC: Canine retinopathies III. The other breeds. J Small Anim Pract 6:185, 1965.

4.   Parry HB: Degenerations of the dog retina   VI. CPRA with pigment epithelial dystrophy. Br J Ophthalmol 38:653, 1954.

5.   Gelatt KN: Cataracts in the Golden retriever. VM/SAC 67:1113, 1972.

6.   Rubin LF: Cataracts in Golden retrievers. J Am Vet Med Assoc 165:457, 1974.

7.   Curtis R: Hereditary cataract in the Golden and Labrador retrievers in the United Kingdom. Trans Am Coll Vet Ophthal 17:23, 1986.

GORDON SETTER

	DISORDER	INHERITANCE	REFERENCE	BREEDING ADVICE
A.	Cataract	Not defined	1	NO
B.	Dry eye	Not defined	2	NO
C.	Entropion/ macroblepharon	Not defined	1,3,4	NO
D.	Progressive Retinal Atrophy	Not defined	4,5,6	NO

Description and Comments

A.   Cataract

Lens opacity which may affect one or both eyes and may involve the lens partially or completely. In cases where cataracts are complete and affect both eyes, blindness results. The prudent approach is to assume cataracts to be hereditary except in cases known to be associated with trauma, other causes of ocular inflammation, specific metabolic diseases, persistent pupillary membranes, persistent hyaloid or nutritional deficiencies.

B.   Dry eye

An abnormality of the tear film, most commonly a deficiency of the aqueous portion, although the mucin and/or lipid layers may be affected; results in ocular irritation and/or vision impairment.

C.   Entropion / macroblepharon

A conformational defect resulting in an "in-rolling" of one or more of the eyelids which may cause ocular irritation. It is likely that entropion is influenced by several genes (polygenic), defining the skin and other structures which make up the eyelids, the amount and weight of the skin covering the head and face, the orbital contents, and the conformation of the skull.

In the Gordon setter, ectropion may be associated with an exceptionally large palpebral fissure and laxity of the canthal structures. Central lower lid ectropion or entropion is then associated with entropion of the adjacent lid. This causes severe ocular irritation.

D.   Progressive Retinal Atrophy (PRA)

A degenerative disease of the retinal visual cells which progresses to blindness. This abnormality may be detected by electroretinogram before it is apparent clinically. In all breeds studied to date, PRA is recessively inherited.

References

1.   Rubin LF: Inherited Eye Diseases in Purebred Dogs. Williams and Wilkins, Baltimore, 1989.

2.   ACVO Genetics Committee, 1992 and/or Data from CERF All-Breeds Report, 1991.

3.   Blogg JR: The Eye in Veterinary Practice. Extraocular Disease. W B Saunders Co, Philadelphia, 1980.

4.   Wyman M: Manual of Small Animal Ophthalmology. Churchill Livingstone, New York, 1986.

5.   Magnusson H: Om nattblindhet hos hund sasom foljd afslaktkapsafvel (On night blindness in the dog following inbreeding). Svensk Vet Tidskr 14:462, 1909.

6.   Mangusson H: Uber retinites pigmentosa und konsanguinitat beim hunde (On retinitis pigmentosa and consanguinity in dogs). Arch Vergl Ophtalmol 2:147, 1911.

7.   Magnusson H: Noch ein fall von nachtblindheit beim hunde (Another case of night blindness in the dog). Graefes Arch Ophthal 93:404, 1917.

GREAT DANE

	DISORDER	INHERITANCE	REFERENCE	BREEDING ADVICE
A.	Entropion	Not defined	--	Breeder option
B.	Ectropion	Not defined	--	Breeder option
C.	Everted cartilage of third eyelid	Not defined	--	Breeder option
D.	Cataract	Not defined	1	NO
E.	Abnormalities associated with partial albinism	Autosomal dominant	2	NO
F.	Progressive Retinal Atrophy	Not defined	--	NO
G.	Glaucoma	Not defined	--	NO

Description and Comments

A. Entropion

A conformational defect resulting in an "in-rolling" of one or more of the eyelids which may cause ocular irritation. It is likely that entropion is influenced by several genes (polygenic), defining the skin and other structures which make up the eyelids, the amount and weight of the skin covering the head and face, the orbital contents, and the conformation of the skull. Entropion and ectropion often occur together in this breed, associated with an abnormally large palpebral fissure.

B. Ectropion

A conformational defect resulting in eversion of the eyelids which may cause ocular irritation. It is likely that ectropion is influenced by several genes (polygenic) defining the skin and other structures which make up the eyelids, the amount and weight of the skin covering the head and face, the orbital contents and the conformation of the skull.

C.   Eversion of the cartilage of the third eyelid

A scroll-like curling of the cartilage of the third eyelid, usually everting the margin. This condition may occur in one or both eyes and may cause mild ocular irritation.

D.   Cataract

Lens opacity which may affect one or both eyes and may involve the lens partially or completely.   In cases where cataracts are complete and affect both eyes, blindness results.   The prudent approach is to assume cataracts to be hereditary except in cases known to be associated with trauma, other causes of ocular inflammation, specific metabolic diseases, persistent pupillary membranes, persistent hyaloid or nutritional deficiencies.   The mode of inheritance in this breed has not been determined.

E.   Abnormalities associated with partial albinism

Multiple ocular defects are seen associated with partial albinism and deafness in Great Danes.   The abnormalities are thought to stem from a common developmental defect.   Ocular defects are anterior segment dysgenesis, equatorial staphylomas, microphthalmia, cortical cataracts, lens luxation, spherophakia, iris coloboma, and blue irides. An autosomal dominant mode of inheritance is suspected. The hearing loss is attributable to cochlea-saccular degeneration.

F.   Progressive Retinal Atrophy (PRA)

A degenerative disease of the retinal visual cells which progresses to blindness.   This abnormality may be detected by electroretinogram before it is apparent clinically.   In all breeds studied to date, PRA is recessively inherited.

G.   Glaucoma

An elevation of intraocular pressure (IOP) which, when sustained, causes intraocular damage resulting in blindness. The elevated IOP occurs because the fluid cannot leave through the iridocorneal angle.   Diagnosis and classification of glaucoma requires measurement of IOP (tonometry) and examination of the iridocorneal angle (gonioscopy). Neither of these tests are part of a routine breed eye screening exam.

References

There are no references providing detailed descriptions of hereditary ocular conditions of the Great Dane breed. The conditions listed above are generally recognized to exist in this breed, as evidenced by repeated references made in general texts.

1.   ACVO Genetics Committee, 1992 and/or Data from CERF All-Breeds Report, 1991.

2.   Gwin RM et al: Multiple ocular defects associated with partial albinism and deafness in the dog. J Am Anim Hosp Assoc 17:401, 1981.

GREAT PYRENEES

	DISORDER	INHERITANCE	REFERENCE	BREEDING ADVICE
A.	Entropion	Not defined	1	Breeder option
B.	Ectropion	Not defined	1	Breeder option
C.	Progressive Retinal Atrophy	Not defined	1	NO

Description and Comments

A.   Entropion

A conformational defect resulting in an "in-rolling" of one or more of the eyelids which may cause ocular irritation. It is likely that entropion is influenced by several genes (polygenic), defining the skin and other structures which make up the eyelids, the amount and weight of the skin covering the head and face, the orbital contents, and the conformation of the skull.

The conformational defect in the Great Pyrenees may result in a vertical shaped palpebral fissure causing a "pagoda" appearance. It can be observed as early as 5 months to 1.5 years of age and surgical correction in this breed is normally required.

B.   Ectropion

A conformational defect resulting in eversion of the eyelids which may cause ocular irritation due to exposure. It is likely that ectropion is influenced by several genes (polygenic) defining the skin and other structures which make up the eyelids, the amount and weight of the skin covering the head and face, the orbital contents and the conformation of the skull.

C.   Progressive Retinal Atrophy (PRA)

A degenerative disease of the retinal visual cells which progresses to blindness. This abnormality may be detected by electroretinogram before it is apparent clinically. In all breeds studied to date, PRA is recessively inherited.

References

There are no references providing detailed descriptions of hereditary ocular conditions of the Great Pyrenees breed. The conditions listed above are generally recognized to exist in this breed, as evidenced by repeated references made in general texts.

1.   ACVO Genetics Committee, 1992 and/or Data from CERF All-Breeds Report, 1991.

GREYHOUND

	DISORDER	INHERITANCE	REFERENCE	BREEDING ADVICE
A.	Pannus	Not defined	1	Breeder option
B.	Progressive Retinal Atrophy	Not defined	2	NO

Description and Comments

A.   Pannus / Chronic superficial keratitis

A bilateral disease of the cornea which usually starts as a grayish haze to the ventral or ventrolateral cornea, followed by the formation of a vascularized subepithelial growth that begins to spread toward the central cornea; pigmentation follows the vascularization. If severe, vision impairment occurs.

B.   Progressive Retinal Atrophy (PRA)

A degenerative disease of the retinal visual cells which progresses to blindness. This abnormality may be detected by electroretinogram before it is apparent clinically. In all breeds studied to date, PRA is recessively inherited.

References

1.   Dice PF: The cornea, In Gelatt KN (ed): Veterinary Ophthalmology. Lea and Febiger, Philadelphia, 1981, p355.

2.   Slatter DH et al: Retinal degeneration in greyhounds. Aust Vet J 56:106, 1980.

HAVANESE

	DISORDER	INHERITANCE	REFERENCE	BREEDING ADVICE
A.	Cataract	Not defined	1	NO
B.	Progressive Retinal Atrophy	Not defined	--	NO
C.	Retinal detachment	Not defined	1	NO

Description and Comments

A. Cataract

Lens opacity which may affect one or both eyes and may involve the lens partially or completely. In cases where cataracts are complete and affect both eyes, blindness results. The prudent approach is to assume cataracts to be hereditary except in cases known to be associated with trauma, other causes of ocular inflammation, specific metabolic diseases, persistent pupillary membrane, persistent hyaloid or nutritional deficiencies. The exact frequency and significance of cataracts in the breed is not known.

B. Progressive Retinal Atrophy (PRA)

A degenerative disease of the retinal visual cells which progresses to blindness. This abnormality may be detected by electroretinogram before it is apparent clinically. In all breeds studied to date, PRA is recessively inherited. The exact frequency and significance of PRA in the breed is not known.

C. Retinal detachment

The separation of the sensory retina from the underlying tissue. It results in blindness when complete.

158

References

There are no references providing detailed descriptions of hereditary ocular conditions of the Havanese breed. The conditions listed above are generally recognized to exist in this breed, as evidenced by repeated references made in general texts.

1. ACVO Genetics Committee, 1992 and/or Data from CERF All-Breeds Report, 1991.

IBIZAN HOUND

	DISORDER	INHERITANCE	REFERENCE	BREEDING ADVICE
A.	Cataract	Not defined	1	NO

Description and Comments

A.   Cataract

Lens opacity which may affect one or both eyes and may involve the lens partially or completely. In cases where cataracts are complete and affect both eyes, blindness results. The prudent approach is to assume cataracts to be hereditary except in cases known to be associated with trauma, other causes of ocular inflammation, specific metabolic diseases, persistent pupillary membrane, persistent hyaloid or nutritional deficiencies.

References

There are no references providing detailed descriptions of hereditary ocular conditions of the Ibizan Hound breed. The conditions listed above are generally recognized to exist in this breed, as evidenced by repeated references made in general texts.

1.   ACVO Genetics Committee, 1992 and/or Data from CERF All-Breeds Report, 1991.

IRISH SETTER

	DISORDER	INHERITANCE	REFERENCE	BREEDING ADVICE
A.	Entropion	Not defined	5	Breeder option
B.	Cataract	Not defined	4	NO
C.	Progressive Retinal Atrophy	Autosomal recessive	1-4	NO

Description and Comments

A.   Entropion

A conformational defect resulting in an "in-rolling" of one or more of the eyelids which may cause ocular irritation. It is likely that entropion is influenced by several genes (polygenic), defining the skin and other structures which make up the eyelids, the amount and weight of the skin covering the head and face, the orbital contents, and the conformation of the skull. In the Irish Setter, the entropion usually involves the lower eyelids.

B.   Cataract

Lens opacity which may affect one or both eyes and may involve the lens partially or completely. In cases where cataracts are complete and affect both eyes, blindness results. The prudent approach is to assume cataracts to be hereditary except in cases known to be associated with trauma, other causes of ocular inflammation, specific metabolic diseases, persistent pupillary membranes, persistent hyaloid or nutritional deficiencies.

C.   Progressive Retinal Atrophy (PRA)

A degenerative disease of the retinal visual cells which progresses to blindness. This abnormality may be detected by electroretinogram before it is apparent clinically. In all breeds studied to date, PRA is recessively inherited.

In the Irish Setter there appears to be more than one form of PRA: 1) rod-cone dysplasia, which can often be clinically observed between 3-12 months of age and as early as 24 days with the ERG. Histologically the disease can be detected by 6 weeks. 2) A later form of progressive retinal atrophy has been observed by several ophthalmologists at 4-5 years of age. The cases in this category that we have observed appear to advance more rapidly than those with rod-cone dysplasia.

Other Conditions Under Consideration

D.   Eversion of the cartilage of the third eyelid

A scroll-like curling of the cartilage of the third eyelid, usually everting the margin. This condition may occur in one or both eyes and may cause mild ocular irritation.

E.   Persistent pupillary membranes (PPM)

Persistent blood vessel remnants in the anterior chamber of the eye which fail to regress normally in the neonatal period. These strands may bridge from iris to iris, iris to cornea, iris to lens, or form sheets of tissue in the anterior chamber. The last three forms pose the greatest threat to vision and when severe, vision impairment or blindness may occur.

F.   Distichiasis

Eyelashes abnormally located in the eyelid margin which may cause ocular irritation. Distichiasis may occur at any time in the life of a dog. It is difficult to make a strong recommendation with regard to breeding dogs with this entity. The hereditary basis has not been established, although it seems probable due to the high incidence in some breeds. Reducing the incidence is a logical goal. When diagnosed, distichiasis should be recorded; breeding discretion is advised.

G.   Persistent hyperplastic primary vitreous (PHPV)

A congenital defect resulting from abnormalities in the development and regression of the hyaloid artery (the primary vitreous) and the interaction of this blood vessel with the posterior lens capsule/cortex during embryogenesis.

References

1.   Hodgman SS et al: Progressive retinal atrophy in dogs I. The disease of Irish Setters (red). Vet Rec 61:185, 1949.

2.   Parry HB: Degenerations of dog retina II. Progressive retinal atrophy of hereditary origin. Br J Ophthalmol 37:487, 1953.

3.   Aguirre GD, Rubin LF: Rod-cone dysplasia (progressive retinal atrophy) in Irish setters. J Am Vet Med Assoc 166:157, 1975.

4.   Rubin LF: <u>Inherited Eye Diseases in Purebred Dogs</u>. Williams and Wilkins, Baltimore, 1989, p169.

5.   ACVO Genetics Committee, 1992 and/or Data from CERF All-Breeds Report, 1991.

IRISH TERRIER

	DISORDER	INHERITANCE	REFERENCE	BREEDING ADVICE
A.	Progressive Retinal Atrophy	Autosomal recessive	1	NO

Description and Comments

A.   Progressive Retinal Atrophy (PRA)

A degenerative disease of the retinal visual cells which progresses to blindness. This abnormality may be detected by electroretinogram before it is apparent clinically. In all breeds studied to date, PRA is recessively inherited.

References

There are no references providing detailed descriptions of hereditary ocular conditions of the Irish Terrier breed. The conditions listed above are generally recognized to exist in this breed, as evidenced by repeated references made in general texts.

1.   ACVO Genetics Committee, 1992 and/or Data from CERF All-Breeds Report, 1991.

IRISH WATER SPANIEL

	DISORDER	INHERITANCE	REFERENCE	BREEDING ADVICE
A.	Cataract	Not defined	1	NO
B.	Progressive Retinal Atrophy	Not defined	1	NO

Description and Comments

A. Cataract

Lens opacity which may affect one or both eyes and may involve the lens partially or completely. In cases where cataracts are complete and affect both eyes, blindness results. The prudent approach is to assume cataracts to be hereditary except in cases known to be associated with trauma, other causes of ocular inflammation, specific metabolic diseases, persistent pupillary membranes, persistent hyaloid or nutritional deficiencies.

B. Progressive Retinal Atrophy (PRA)

A degenerative disease of the retinal visual cells which progresses to blindness. This abnormality may be detected by electroretinogram before it is apparent clinically. In all breeds studied to date, PRA is recessively inherited.

References

There are no references providing detailed descriptions of hereditary ocular conditions of the Irish Water Spaniel breed. The conditions listed above are generally recognized to exist in this breed, as evidenced by repeated references made in general texts.

1. ACVO Genetics Committee, 1992 and/or Data from CERF All-Breeds Report, 1991.

IRISH WOLFHOUND

	DISORDER	INHERITANCE	REFERENCE	BREEDING ADVICE
A.	Entropion	Not defined	1	Breeder option
B.	Cataract	Not defined	1	NO
C.	Everted cartilage of third eyelid	Not defined	1	Breeder option

Description and Comments

A. Entropion

A conformational defect resulting in an "in-rolling" of one or more of the eyelids which may cause ocular irritation. It is likely that entropion is influenced by several genes (polygenic), defining the skin and other structures which make up the eyelids, the amount and weight of the skin covering the head and face, the orbital contents, and the conformation of the skull.

B. Cataract

Lens opacity which may affect one or both eyes and may involve the lens partially or completely. In cases where cataracts are complete and affect both eyes, blindness results. The prudent approach is to assume cataracts to be hereditary except in cases known to be associated with trauma, other causes of ocular inflammation, specific metabolic diseases, persistent pupillary membranes, persistent hyaloid or nutritional deficiencies.

C. Eversion of the cartilage of the third eyelid

A scroll-like curling of the cartilage of the third eyelid, usually everting the margin. This condition may occur in one or both eyes and may cause mild ocular irritation.

References

There are no references providing detailed descriptions of hereditary ocular conditions of the Irish Wolfhound breed. The conditions listed above are generally recognized to exist in this breed, as evidenced by repeated references made in general texts.

1.   ACVO Genetics Committee, 1992 and/or Data from CERF All-Breeds Report, 1991.

ITALIAN GREYHOUND

	DISORDER	INHERITANCE	REFERENCE	BREEDING ADVICE
A.	Cataract	Not defined	1	NO
B.	Glaucoma	Not defined	2	NO
C.	Vitreal degeneration	Not defined	2	Breeder Option
D.	Progressive Retinal Atrophy	Not defined	1,2	NO

Description and Comments

A.   Cataract

Lens opacity which may affect one or both eyes and may involve the lens partially or completely. In cases where cataracts are complete and affect both eyes, blindness results. The prudent approach is to assume cataracts to be hereditary except in cases known to be associated with trauma, other causes of ocular inflammation, specific metabolic diseases, persistent pupillary membrane, persistent hyaloid or nutritional deficiencies.

In the Italian Greyhound, posterior subcapsular and cortical cataracts at two to three years of age appear to be the more common location of occurrence, with progression noted in an undetermined percentage of dogs.

B.   Glaucoma

An elevation of intraocular pressure (IOP) which, when sustained, causes intraocular damage resulting in blindness. The elevated IOP occurs because the fluid cannot leave through the iridocorneal angle. Diagnosis and classification of glaucoma requires measurement of IOP (tonometry) and examination of the iridocorneal angle (gonioscopy). Neither of these tests are part of a routine breed eye screening exam.

168

In the Italian Greyhound, degeneration of the vitreous may play a predominant role in the development of glaucoma as there is definite anterior displacement of vitreous observed in some glaucoma cases.

C.   Vitreal degeneration

A liquefaction of the vitreous gel which may predispose to retinal detachment and/or glaucoma. In the Italian Greyhound, glaucoma appears to be more interrelated than retinal detachment.

D.   Progressive Retinal Atrophy (PRA)

A degenerative disease of the retinal visual cells which progresses to blindness. This abnormality may be detected by electroretinogram before it is apparent clinically. In all breeds studied to date, PRA is recessively inherited.

Progressive retinal atrophy in the Italian Greyhound is relatively uncommon. It has been observed in dogs in the advanced stage by four to five years of age.

References

1.   Rubin, LF: Inherited Eye Diseases in Purebred Dogs. William and Wilkins, Baltimore, 1989, p177-178.

2.   ACVO Genetics Committee, 1992 and/or Data from CERF All-Breeds Report, 1991.

JACK RUSSELL TERRIER

	DISORDER	INHERITANCE	REFERENCE	BREEDING ADVICE
A.	Lens luxation	Not defined	1-3	NO

Description and Comments

A.   Lens luxation

Partial (subluxation) or complete displacement of the lens from its normal anatomic site behind the pupil. Lens luxation not associated with trauma or inflammation is presumed to be inherited. Lens luxation may result in elevated intraocular pressure (glaucoma) causing vision impairment or blindness.

References

1. Lawson DD: Luxation of the crystalline lens in the dog. J Sm Anim Pract 10:461, 1969.

2. Curtis R, Barnett KC: Primary lens luxation in the dog. J Sm Anim Pract 21:657, 1980.

3. Curtis R, Barnett KC, Lewis SJ: Clinical and pathological observations concerning the aetiology of primary lens luxation in the dog. Vet Rec 112:238, 1983.

JAPANESE CHIN

	DISORDER	INHERITANCE	REFERENCE	BREEDING ADVICE
A.	Cataract	Not defined	1	NO
B.	Distichiasis	Not defined	1	Breeder option
C.	Progressive Retinal Atrophy	Not defined	1	NO

Description and Comments

A.   Cataract

Lens opacity which may affect one or both eyes and may involve the lens partially or completely. In cases where cataracts are complete and affect both eyes, blindness results. The prudent approach is to assume cataracts to be hereditary except in cases known to be associated with trauma, other causes of ocular inflammation, specific metabolic diseases, persistent pupillary membranes, persistent hyaloid or nutritional deficiencies.

B.   Distichiasis

Eyelashes abnormally located in the eyelid margin which may cause ocular irritation. Distichiasis may occur at any time in the life of a dog. It is difficult to make a strong recommendation with regard to breeding dogs with this entity. The hereditary basis has not been established, although it seems probable due to the high incidence in some breeds. Reducing the incidence is a logical goal. When diagnosed, distichiasis should be recorded; breeding discretion is advised.

B.   Progressive Retinal Atrophy (PRA)

A degenerative disease of the retinal visual cells which progresses to blindness. This abnormality may be detected by electroretinogram before it is apparent clinically. In all breeds studied to date, PRA is recessively inherited.

References

There are no references providing detailed descriptions of hereditary ocular conditions of the Japanese Chin breed. The conditions listed above are generally recognized to exist in this breed, as evidenced by repeated references made in general texts.

1.   ACVO Genetics Committee, 1992 and/or Data from CERF All-Breeds Report, 1991.

KEESHOUND

	DISORDER	INHERITANCE	REFERENCE	BREEDING ADVICE
A.	Cataract	Not defined	1	NO
B.	Central Progressive Retinal Atrophy	Not defined	2	NO
C.	Progressive Retinal Atrophy	Not defined	1	NO
D.	Glaucoma	Not defined	1	NO

Description and Comments

A. Cataract

Lens opacity which may affect one or both eyes and may involve the lens partially or completely. In cases where cataracts are complete and affect both eyes, blindness results. The prudent approach is to assume cataracts to be hereditary except in cases known to be associated with trauma, other causes of ocular inflammation, specific metabolic diseases, persistent pupillary membranes, persistent hyaloid or nutritional deficiencies.

B. Central Progressive Retinal Atrophy (CPRA)

A progressive retinal degeneration in which photoreceptor death occurs secondary to disease of the underlying pigment epithelium. Progression is slow and some animals never lose vision. CPRA occurs in England, but is uncommon elsewhere.

C. Progressive Retinal Atrophy (PRA)

A degenerative disease of the retinal visual cells which progresses to blindness. This abnormality may be detected by electroretinogram before it is apparent clinically. In all breeds studied to date, PRA is recessively inherited.

D.   Glaucoma

An elevation of intraocular pressure (IOP) which, when sustained, causes intraocular damage resulting in blindness. The elevated IOP occurs because the fluid cannot leave through the iridocorneal angle. Diagnosis and classification of glaucoma requires measurement of IOP (tonometry) and examination of the iridocorneal angle (gonioscopy). Neither of these tests are part of a routine breed eye screening exam.

References

There are no references providing detailed descriptions of hereditary ocular conditions of the Keeshound breed. The conditions listed above are generally recognized to exist in this breed, as evidenced by repeated references made in general texts.

1.   ACVO Genetics Committee, 1992 and/or Data from CERF All-Breeds Report, 1991.

2.   Whitley RD, Miller TR: Predisposition to ocular disease in dogs. Proc CAVO and ASVO Joint Meeting in conjunction with the 23rd World Veterinary Congress, 1987, p20.

KERRY BLUE TERRIER

	DISORDER	INHERITANCE	REFERENCE	BREEDING ADVICE
A.	Entropion	Not defined	--	Breeder option
B.	Cataract	Not defined	--	NO
C.	Progressive Retinal Atrophy	Not defined	--	NO

Description and Comments

A.   Entropion

A conformational defect resulting in an "in-rolling" of one or more of the eyelids which may cause ocular irritation. It is likely that entropion is influenced by several genes (polygenic), defining the skin and other structures which make up the eyelids, the amount and weight of the skin covering the head and face, the orbital contents, and the conformation of the skull.

B.   Cataract

Lens opacity which may affect one or both eyes and may involve the lens partially or completely. In cases where cataracts are complete and affect both eyes, blindness results. The prudent approach is to assume cataracts to be hereditary except in cases known to be associated with trauma, other causes of ocular inflammation, specific metabolic diseases, persistent pupillary membranes, persistent hyaloid or nutritional deficiencies.

C.   Progressive Retinal Atrophy (PRA)

A degenerative disease of the retinal visual cells which progresses to blindness. This abnormality may be detected by electroretinogram before it is apparent clinically. In all breeds studied to date, PRA is recessively inherited.

References

There are no references providing detailed descriptions of hereditary ocular conditions of the Kerry Blue Terrier breed. The conditions listed above are generally recognized to exist in this breed, as evidenced by repeated references made in general texts.

1.   ACVO Genetics Committee, 1992 and/or Data from CERF All-Breeds Report, 1991.

KOMONDOR

	DISORDER	INHERITANCE	REFERENCE	BREEDING ADVICE
A.	Entropion	Not defined	--	NO
B.	Cataract	Not defined	--	NO

Description and Comments

A.   Entropion

A conformational defect resulting in an "in-rolling" of one or more of the eyelids which may cause ocular irritation. It is likely that entropion is influenced by several genes (polygenic), defining the skin and other structures which make up the eyelids, the amount and weight of the skin covering the head and face, the orbital contents, and the conformation of the skull.

B.   Cataract

Lens opacity which may affect one or both eyes and may involve the lens partially or completely. In cases where cataracts are complete and affect both eyes, blindness results. The prudent approach is to assume cataracts to be hereditary except in cases known to be associated with trauma, other causes of ocular inflammation, specific metabolic diseases, persistent pupillary membrane, persistent hyaloid or nutritional deficiencies.

Other Conditions Under Consideration

C.   Ectropion

A conformational defect resulting in eversion of the eyelids which may cause ocular irritation. It is likely that ectropion is influenced by several genes (polygenic) defining the skin and other structures which make up the eyelids, the amount and weight of the skin covering the head and face, the orbital contents and the conformation of the skull.

D.   Distichiasis

Eyelashes abnormally located in the eyelid margin which may cause ocular irritation. Distichiasis may occur at any time in the life of a dog. It is difficult to make a strong recommendation with regard to breeding dogs with this entity. The hereditary basis has not been established although it seems probable due to the high incidence in some breeds. Reducing the incidence is a logical goal. When diagnosed, distichiasis should be recorded; breeding discretion is advised.

E.   Prolapse of the gland of the third eyelid

A protrusion of the tear gland associated with the third eyelid. The mode of inheritance of this disorder is unknown. The exposed gland may become irritated. Commonly referred to as "cherry eye".

F.   Eversion of the cartilage of the third eyelid

A scroll-like curling of the cartilage of the third eyelid, usually everting the margin. This condition may occur in one or both eyes and may cause mild ocular irritation.

References

There are no references providing detailed descriptions of hereditary ocular conditions of the Komondor breed. The conditions listed above are generally recognized to exist in this breed, as evidenced by repeated references made in general texts.

1.   ACVO Genetics Committee, 1992 and/or Data from CERF All-Breeds Report, 1991.

KUVASZ

	DISORDER	INHERITANCE	REFERENCE	BREEDING ADVICE
A.	Entropion	Not defined	--	Breeder option

Description and Comments

A. Entropion

A conformational defect resulting in an "in-rolling" of one or more of the eyelids which may cause ocular irritation. It is likely that entropion is influenced by several genes (polygenic), defining the skin and other structures which make up the eyelids, the amount and weight of the skin covering the head and face, the orbital contents, and the conformation of the skull.

Other Conditions Under Consideration

B. Ectropion

A conformational defect resulting in eversion of the eyelids which may cause ocular irritation. It is likely that ectropion is influenced by several genes (polygenic) defining the skin and other structures which make up the eyelids, the amount and weight of the skin covering the head and face, the orbital contents and the conformation of the skull.

C. Distichiasis

Eyelashes abnormally located in the eyelid margin which may cause ocular irritation. Distichiasis may occur at any time in the life of a dog. It is difficult to make a strong recommendation with regard to breeding dogs with this entity. The hereditary basis has not been established although it seems probable due to the high incidence in some breeds. Reducing the incidence is a logical goal. When diagnosed, distichiasis should be recorded; breeding discretion is advised.

D.   Prolapse of the gland of the third eyelid

A protrusion of the tear gland associated with the third eyelid. The mode of inheritance of this disorder is unknown. The exposed gland may become irritated. Commonly referred to as "cherry eye".

E.   Eversion of the cartilage of the third eyelid

A scroll-like curling of the cartilage of the third eyelid, usually everting the margin. This condition may occur in one or both eyes and may cause mild ocular irritation. The mode of inheritance is unknown.

F.   Cataract

Lens opacity which may affect one or both eyes and may involve the lens partially or completely. In cases where cataracts are complete and affect both eyes, blindness results. The prudent approach is to assume cataracts to be hereditary except in cases known to be associated with trauma, other causes of ocular inflammation, specific metabolic diseases, persistent pupillary membranes, persistent hyaloid or nutritional deficiencies.

References

There are no references providing detailed descriptions of hereditary ocular conditions of the Kuvasz breed. The conditions listed above are generally recognized to exist in this breed, as evidenced by repeated references made in general texts.

1.   ACVO Genetics Committee, 1992 and/or Data from CERF All-Breeds Report, 1991.

LABRADOR RETRIEVER

	DISORDER	INHERITANCE	REFERENCE	BREEDING ADVICE
A.	Entropion	Not defined	--	Breeder option
B.	Distichiasis	Not defined	1	Breeder option
C.	Cataract	Dominant with incomplete penetrance	2	NO
D.	Progressive Retinal Atrophy	Autosomal recessive	3,4	NO
E.	Central Progressive Retinal Atrophy	Not defined	5	NO
F.	Retinal dysplasia - detachment	Autosomal recessive	6,7	NO
G.	Retinal dysplasia - focal/geographic/ detachment (with skeletal defects)	Incompletely dominant	8-10	NO

Description and Comments

A.   Entropion

A conformational defect resulting in an "in-rolling" of one or more of the eyelids which may cause ocular irritation. It is likely that entropion is influenced by several genes (polygenic), defining the skin and other structures which make up the eyelids, the amount and weight of the skin covering the head and face, the orbital contents, and the conformation of the skull. Selection should be directed against entropion and toward a head conformation that reduces or eliminates the likelihood of the defect.

B. Distichiasis

Eyelashes abnormally located in the eyelid margin which may cause ocular irritation. Distichiasis may occur at any time in the life of a dog. It is difficult to make a strong recommendation with regard to breeding dogs with this entity. The hereditary basis has not been established, although it seems probable due to the high incidence in some breeds. Reducing the incidence is a logical goal. When diagnosed, distichiasis should be recorded; breeding discretion is advised.

C. Cataract

Lens opacity which may affect one or both eyes and may involve the lens partially or completely. In cases where cataracts are complete and affect both eyes, blindness results. The prudent approach is to assume cataracts to be hereditary except in cases known to be associated with trauma, other causes of ocular inflammation, specific metabolic diseases, persistent pupillary membranes, persistent hyaloid or nutritional deficiencies.

The most frequently reported cataracts in the breed are bilateral or unilateral, focal, posterior polar (posterior cortical)/subcapsular cataracts usually present between 1-3 years of age. These are generally stationary or very slowly progressive and generally do not interfere with vision. It has been suggested that these cataracts are inherited as dominant with incomplete penetrance, but definitive breeding studies are still required to verify this hypothesis.

A second type of cataract is a progressive cortical cataract which may involve the entire lens. It is not clear whether this is a distinct entity, or an aberrant form of the posterior polar cataract.

D. Progressive Retinal Atrophy (PRA)

A degenerative disease of the retinal visual cells which progresses to blindness. This abnormality may be detected by electroretinogram before it is apparent clinically. In all breeds studied to date, PRA is recessively inherited.

In the Labrador retriever, early fundus abnormalities usually appear after 4 years of age. The electroretinogram (ERG) shows marked functional abnormalities indicative of a progressive rod-cone degeneration. The age for early diagnosis by ERG is after 18 months of age. Studies have shown that PRA in the Labrador retriever is inherited as autosomal recessive. The mutation is allelic to that present in miniature poodles and English/American cocker spaniels and the gene locus is termed progressive rod-cone degeneration (*prcd*).

E.   Central Progressive Retinal Atrophy (CPRA)

A progressive retinal degeneration in which photoreceptor death occurs secondary to disease of the underlying pigment epithelium. Progression is slow and some animals never lose vision. CPRA occurs in England, but is uncommon elsewhere.

The lesions first appear in the posterior pole (central retina), enlarge, coalesce and result in secondary retinal atrophy; progression from the posterior pole to the periphery occurs later. The age of onset varies from young adults to older animals but usually before 5 years of age. Although reported to be dominant with incomplete penetrance, the mode of inheritance of CPRA remains undetermined. The disease has rarely been seen in dogs bred and raised in the U.S. This limited geographic distribution has led some to speculate about a nutritional basis.

F.   Retinal dysplasia

Abnormal development of the retina present at birth and recognized to have three forms:

1) Retinal dysplasia - **folds**: linear, triangular, curved or curvilinear foci of retinal folding that may be single or multiple.
2) Retinal dysplasia - **geographic**: any irregularly shaped area of abnormal retinal development, representing changes not accountable by simple folding.
3) Retinal dysplasia - **detachment**: either of the above described forms of retinal dysplasia associated with separation (detachment) of the retina.

The two latter forms are associated with vision impairment or blindness. Retinal dysplasia is known to be inherited in many breeds. The genetic relationship between the three forms of the disease is not known for all breeds.

In the Labrador retriever the defect is inherited as autosomal recessive and results in early retinal detachment and blindness. Lens and corneal opacities can also be present, but skeletal abnormalities (see below) are not present. The condition of generalized retinal dysplasia without skeletal abnormalities has been reported primarily in Europe, and is rarely if ever seen in the United States.

G.   Retinal dysplasia - focal/geographic/detachment (with skeletal defects)

An inherited defect of the Labrador retriever which can affect both the eye and the forelimbs. The gene has recessive effects on the skeleton and incompletely dominant effects on the eye. Dogs homozygous recessive for the gene defect have retinal dysplasia (detachment), cataracts and corneal pigmentation, associated with abnormalities of the appendicular skeleton (a form of short-limbed dwarfism). The ocular abnormalities result in blindness in most dogs. Heterozygous dogs have a bilateral/unilateral congenital retinal defect resulting in ophthalmoscopically visible retinal dysplasia (folds and/or geographic lesions) present in the central tapetal region near the major retinal vessels. Vision can be normal to impaired. The condition in the heterozygous dog is stationary although, in rare cases, progressive retinal detachments have developed. The term "incompletely dominant" in regard to the ocular lesions refers to the difference in phenotype between the homozygous and heterozygous state. This condition has been found primarily in field trial lines.

Other Conditions Under Consideration

H.   Corneal dystrophy

A non-inflammatory corneal opacity (white to gray) present in one or more of the corneal layers; usually inherited and bilateral.

I.   Persistent hyaloid artery (PHA)

A congenital defect resulting from abnormalities in the development and regression of the hyaloid artery. The blood vessel can be present in the vitreous body as a small vascular strand (PHA) or as a non-vascularized strand that appears gray-white (persistent hyaloid remnant).

J.   Persistent hyperplastic primary vitreous / persistent tunica vasculosa lentis (PHPV/PTVL)

A congenital defect resulting from abnormalities in the development and regression of the hyaloid artery (the primary vitreous) and the interaction of this blood vessel with the posterior lens capsule/cortex during embryogenesis. This condition is often associated with **persistent tunica vasculosa lentis (PTVL)** which results from failure of regression of the embryologic vascular network which surrounds the developing lens.

The majority of affected dogs have a retrolental fibrovascular plaque and variable lenticular defects which include posterior lenticonus/globus, colobomata, intralenticular hemorrhage and/or secondary cataracts. Vision impairment may result.

References

1.   ACVO Genetics Committee, 1992 and/or Data from CERF All-Breeds Report, 1991.

2.   Curtis R, Barnett KC: A survey of cataracts in Golden and Labrador retrievers. J Sm Anim Pract 30:277, 1989.

3. Aguirre GD, Acland GM: Variation in retinal degeneration phenotype inherited at the *prcd* locus. Exp Eye Res 46:663, 1988.

4. Aguirre GD, Acland GM: Inherited retinal degeneration in the Labrador retriever dog. A new animal model of RP? Invest Ophthalmol Vis Sci (Supp) 32(4), 1991.

5. Hereditary eye abnormalities in the dog #2. Central progressive retinal atrophy. The Animal Health Trust, Small Animals Centre. November, 1977.

6. Barnett KC et al: Hereditary retinal dysplasia in the Labrador retriever in England and Sweden. J Small Anim Pract 10:755, 1970.

7. Kock E: Retinal dysplasia. Thesis, Stockholm, 1974.

8. Carrig CB et al: Retinal dysplasia associated with skeletal abnormalities in Labrador retrievers. J Am Vet Med Assoc 170:49, 1974.

9. Nelson D, MacMillan A: Multifocal retinal dysplasia in the field trial Labrador retriever. J Am Anim Hosp Assoc 19:388, 1983.

10. Carrig CB et al: Inheritance of associated ocular and skeletal dysplasia in Labrador retrievers. J Am Vet Med Assoc 193:1269, 1988.

LHASA APSO

	DISORDER	INHERITANCE	REFERENCE	BREEDING ADVICE
A.	Distichiasis	Not defined	1	Breeder option
B.	Entropion	Not defined	1	Breeder option
C.	Ectopic cilia	Not defined	1	Breeder option
D.	Dry eye	Not defined	1	NO
E.	Progressive Retinal Atrophy	Not defined	1	NO
F.	Cataract	Not defined	1	NO
G.	Prolapsed gland of third eyelid	Not defined	1	Breeder option
H.	Exposure keratopathy	Not defined	1	NO

Description and Comments

A. Distichiasis

Eyelashes abnormally located in the eyelid margin which may cause ocular irritation. Distichiasis may occur at any time in the life of a dog. It is difficult to make a strong recommendation with regard to breeding dogs with this entity. The hereditary basis has not been established although it seems probable due to the high incidence in some breeds. Reducing the incidence is a logical goal. When diagnosed, distichiasis should be recorded; breeding discretion is advised.

B. Entropion

A conformational defect resulting in an "in-rolling" of one or more of the eyelids which may cause ocular irritation. It is likely that entropion is influenced by several genes (polygenic), defining the skin and other structures which make up the eyelids, the amount and weight of the skin covering the head and face, the orbital contents, and the conformation of the skull. The medial entropion seen in this breed causes an anatomical blockage of the lacrimal puncta and can cause epiphora.

C.   Ectopic cilia

Aberrant hair emerging through the eyelid conjunctiva. Ectopic cilia occur more frequently in younger dogs and cause discomfort and corneal disease.

D.   Dry eye

An abnormality of the tear film, most commonly a deficiency of the aqueous portion, although the mucin and/or lipid layers may be affected; results in ocular irritation and/or vision impairment.

E.   Progressive Retinal Atrophy (PRA)

A degenerative disease of the retinal visual cells which progresses to blindness. This abnormality may be detected by electroretinogram before it is apparent clinically. In all breeds studied to date, PRA is recessively inherited.

F.   Cataract

Lens opacity which may affect one or both eyes and may involve the lens partially or completely. In cases where cataracts are complete and affect both eyes, blindness results. The prudent approach is to assume cataracts to be hereditary except in cases known to be associated with trauma, other causes of ocular inflammation, specific metabolic diseases, persistent pupillary membranes, persistent hyaloid or nutritional deficiencies.

G.   Prolapsed gland of the third eyelid

Protrusion of the tear gland associated with the third eyelid. The mode of inheritance of this disorder is unknown. The exposed gland may become irritated. Commonly referred to as "cherry eye".

H.   Exposure keratopathy syndrome

A corneal disease involving all or part of the cornea, resulting from inadequate blinking. This results from a combination of anatomic features including shallow orbits, exophthalmos, macroblepharon, and lagophthalmos.

Other Conditions Under Consideration

I.   Ciliated caruncle

Fleshy conjunctival tissue at the nasal canthus; may contain hair which, if contacting the cornea, may cause irritation and/or tearing.

References

There are no references providing detailed descriptions of hereditary ocular conditions of the Lhasa Apso breed. The conditions listed above are generally recognized to exist in this breed, as evidenced by repeated references made in general texts.

1.   ACVO Genetics Committee, 1992 and/or Data from CERF All-Breeds Report, 1991.

LOWCHEN

	DISORDER	INHERITANCE	REFERENCE	BREEDING ADVICE
A.	Cataracts	Not defined	1	NO
B.	Progressive Retinal Atrophy	Not defined	1	NO

Description and Comments

A. Cataract

Lens opacity which may affect one or both eyes and may involve the lens partially or completely. In cases where cataracts are complete and affect both eyes, blindness results. The prudent approach is to assume cataracts to be hereditary except in cases known to be associated with trauma, other causes of ocular inflammation, specific metabolic diseases, persistent pupillary membrane, persistent hyaloid or nutritional deficiencies.

B. Progressive Retinal Atrophy (PRA)

A degenerative disease of the retinal visual cells which progresses to blindness. This abnormality may be detected by electroretinogram before it is apparent clinically. In all breeds studied to date, PRA is recessively inherited.

Other Conditions Under Consideration

C. Vitreal degeneration

A liquefaction of the vitreous gel which may predispose to retinal detachment.

References

There are no references providing detailed descriptions of hereditary ocular conditions of the Lowchen breed. The conditions listed above are generally recognized to exist in this breed, as evidenced by repeated references made in general texts.

1. ACVO Genetics Committee, 1992 and/or Data from CERF All-Breeds Report, 1991.

MALTESE

	DISORDER	INHERITANCE	REFERENCE	BREEDING ADVICE
A.	Distichiasis	Not defined	1	Breeder option
B.	Progressive Retinal Atrophy	Not defined	1	NO

Description and Comments

A.   Distichiasis

Eyelashes abnormally located in the eyelid margin which may cause ocular irritation. Distichiasis may occur at any time in the life of a dog. It is difficult to make a strong recommendation with regard to breeding dogs with this entity. The hereditary basis has not been established, although it seems probable due to the high incidence in some breeds. Reducing the incidence is a logical goal. When diagnosed, distichiasis should be recorded; breeding discretion is advised.

B.   Progressive Retinal Atrophy (PRA)

A degenerative disease of the retinal visual cells which progresses to blindness. This abnormality may be detected by electroretinogram before it is apparent clinically. In all breeds studied to date, PRA is recessively inherited.

Other Conditions Under Consideration

C.   Ciliated caruncle

Fleshy conjunctival tissue at the nasal canthus; may contain hair (ciliated caruncle) which, if contacting the cornea, may cause irritation and/or tearing.

References

There are no references providing detailed descriptions of hereditary ocular conditions of the Maltese breed. The conditions listed above are generally recognized to exist in this breed, as evidenced by repeated references made in general texts.

1.   ACVO Genetics Committee, 1992 and/or Data from CERF All-Breeds Report, 1991.

MANCHESTER TERRIER
(Toy and Standard)

	DISORDER	INHERITANCE	REFERENCE	BREEDING ADVICE
A.	Cataract	Not defined	1	NO
B.	Lens luxation	Not defined	1-3	NO
C.	Progressive Retinal Atrophy	Not defined	1	NO

Description and Comments

A. Cataract

Lens opacity which may affect one or both eyes and may involve the lens partially or completely. In cases where cataracts are complete and affect both eyes, blindness results. The prudent approach is to assume cataracts to be hereditary except in cases known to be associated with trauma, other causes of ocular inflammation, specific metabolic diseases, persistent pupillary membranes, persistent hyaloid or nutritional deficiencies.

The exact frequency and significance of cataract in the Manchester terrier is unknown. Complete cataracts are reported in older dogs, although the exact age of onset is unknown.

B. Lens luxation

Partial (subluxation) or complete displacement of the lens from the normal anatomic site. Lens luxation not associated with trauma or inflammation is presumed to be inherited. Lens luxation may result in elevated intraocular pressure (glaucoma) causing vision impairment or blindness.

C. Progressive Retinal Atrophy

A degenerative disease of the retinal visual cells which progresses to blindness. This abnormality may be detected by electroretinogram before it is apparent clinically. In all breeds studied to date, PRA is recessively inherited.

References

There are no references providing detailed descriptions of hereditary ocular conditions of the Manchester Terrier breed. The conditions listed above are generally recognized to exist in this breed, as evidenced by repeated references made in general texts.

1.   ACVO Genetics Committee, 1992 and/or Data from CERF All-Breeds Report, 1991.

2.   Magrane WG: <u>Canine Ophthalmology</u>. 3rd ed. Philadelphia, Lea & Febiger, 1977.

3.   Slatter DH: <u>Fundamentals of Veterinary Ophthalmology.</u>   Philadelphia, W B Saunders, 1981.

MASTIFF

	DISORDER	INHERITANCE	REFERENCE	BREEDING ADVICE
A.	Entropion	Not defined	--	Breeder option
B.	Ectropion	Not defined	--	Breeder option
C.	Macroblepharon	Not defined	--	Breeder option
D.	Persistent pupillary membrane	Not defined	--	Breeder option
E.	Retinal dysplasia - folds	Not defined	--	Breeder option
F.	Progressive Retinal Atrophy	Not defined	--	NO

Description and Comments

A.   Entropion

A conformational defect resulting in an "in-rolling" of one or more of the eyelids which may cause ocular irritation. It is likely that entropion is influenced by several genes (polygenic), defining the skin and other structures which make up the eyelids, the amount and weight of the skin covering the head and face, the orbital contents, and the conformation of the skull.

B.   Ectropion

A conformational defect resulting in eversion of the eyelids, which may cause ocular irritation due to exposure. It is likely that ectropion is influenced by several genes (polygenic), defining the skin and other structures which make up the eyelids, the amount and weight of the skin covering the head and face, the orbital contents and the conformation of the skull.

C.   Macroblepharon

Abnormally large eyelid opening; may lead to secondary conditions associated with corneal exposure.

D.   Persistent pupillary membranes (PPM)

Persistent blood vessel remnants in the anterior chamber of the eye which fail to regress normally in the neonatal period. These strands may bridge from iris to iris, iris to cornea, iris to lens, or form sheets of tissue in the anterior chamber. The last three forms pose the greatest threat to vision and when severe, vision impairment or blindness may occur.

E.   Retinal dysplasia

Abnormal development of the retina present at birth and recognized to have three forms:

1) Retinal dysplasia - **folds**: linear, triangular, curved or curvilinear foci of retinal folding that may be single or multiple.
2) Retinal dysplasia - **geographic**: any irregularly shaped area of abnormal retinal development, representing changes not accountable by simple folding.
3) Retinal dysplasia - **detachment**: either of the above described forms of retinal dysplasia associated with separation (detachment) of the retina.

The two latter forms are associated with vision impairment or blindness. Retinal dysplasia is known to be inherited in many breeds. The genetic relationship between the three forms of the disease is not known for all breeds.

F.   Progressive Retinal Atrophy (PRA)

A degenerative disease of the retinal visual cells which progresses to blindness. This abnormality may be detected by electroretinogram before it is apparent clinically. In all breeds studied to date, PRA is recessively inherited.

Other Conditions Under Consideration

G.   Exposure keratopathy syndrome

A corneal disease involving all or part of the cornea, resulting from a combination of contributing anatomic features including shallow orbits, excessive exophthalmia, macroblepharon and lagophthalmos.

H.   Distichiasis

Eyelashes abnormally located in the eyelid margin which may cause ocular irritation. Distichiasis may occur at any time in the life of a dog. It is difficult to make a strong recommendation with regard to breeding dogs with this entity. The hereditary basis

194

has not been established although it seems probable due to the high incidence in some breeds. Reducing the incidence is a logical goal. When diagnosed, distichiasis should be recorded; breeding discretion is advised.

I.   Prolapse of the gland of the third eyelid

Protrusion of the tear gland associated with the third eyelid. The mode of inheritance of this disorder is unknown. The exposed gland may become irritated. Commonly referred to as "cherry eye".

J.   Eversion of the cartilage of the third eyelid

A scroll-like curling of the cartilage of the third eyelid, usually everting the margin. This condition may occur in one or both eyes and may cause mild ocular irritation. The mode of inheritance is unknown.

K.   Cataract

Lens opacity which may affect one or both eyes and may involve the lens partially or completely. In cases where cataracts are complete and affect both eyes, blindness results. The prudent approach is to assume cataracts to be hereditary except in cases known to be associated with trauma, other causes of ocular inflammation, specific metabolic diseases, persistent pupillary membranes, persistent hyaloid or nutritional deficiencies.

L.   Iris cysts

Pigmented cysts arise from the posterior pigmented epithelial cells of the iris and remain attached or break free, floating as pigmented spheres of various sizes and pigments in the anterior chamber. Some cysts tend to adhere to the posterior surface of the cornea. Rarely, cysts may be numerous enough to impair vision. The mode of inheritance is unknown.

References

There are no references providing detailed descriptions of hereditary ocular conditions of the Mastiff breed. The conditions listed above are generally recognized to exist in this breed, as evidenced by repeated references made in general texts.

1.   ACVO Genetics Committee, 1992 and/or Data from CERF All-Breeds Report, 1991.

MINIATURE BULL TERRIER

	DISORDER	INHERITANCE	REFERENCE	BREEDING ADVICE
A.	Entropion	Not defined	1	Breeder option
B.	Lens luxation	Not defined	2	NO

Description and Comments

A. Entropion

A conformational defect resulting in "in-rolling" of one or more of the eyelids which may cause ocular irritation. It is likely that entropion is influenced by several genes (polygenic), defining the skin and other structures which make up the eyelids, the amount and weight of the skin covering the head and face, the orbital contents and the conformation of the skull.

B. Luxated lens

Partial (subluxation) or complete displacement of the lens from the normal anatomic site behind the pupil. Lens luxation not associated with trauma or inflammation is presumed to be inherited. Lens luxation may result in elevated intraocular pressure (glaucoma) causing vision impairment or blindness.

References

1. ACVO Genetics Committee, 1992 and/or Data from CERF All-Breeds Report, 1991.

2. Curtis R, Barnett KC, Startup FG: Primary lens luxation in the miniature bull terrier. Vet Rec 112: 328, 1983.

MINIATURE PINSCHER

	DISORDER	INHERITANCE	REFERENCE	BREEDING ADVICE
A.	Corneal lipid dystrophy	Not defined	1,3	NO
B.	Cataract	Not defined	1,3	NO
C.	Progressive Retinal Atrophy	Not defined	2	NO

Description and Comments

A.   Corneal dystrophy

A non-inflammatory corneal opacity (white to gray) present in one or more of the corneal layers; usually inherited and bilateral.

B.   Cataract

Lens opacity which may affect one or both eyes and may involve the lens partially or completely. In cases where cataracts are complete and affect both eyes, blindness results. The prudent approach is to assume cataracts to be hereditary except in cases known to be associated with trauma, other causes of ocular inflammation, specific metabolic diseases, persistent pupillary membranes, persistent hyaloid or nutritional deficiencies.

C.   Progressive Retinal Atrophy (PRA)

A degenerative disease of the retinal visual cells which progresses to blindness. This abnormality may be detected by electroretinogram before it is apparent clinically. In all breeds studied to date, PRA is recessively inherited.

References

There are no references providing detailed descriptions of hereditary ocular conditions of the Miniature Pinscher. The conditions listed above are generally recognized to exist in this breed, as evidenced by repeated references made in general texts.

1.   Rubin L: Inherited Eye Diseases in Purebred Dogs. Williams & Wilkins, Baltimore, 1989.

2.   Priester WA: Canine progressive retinal atrophy. Occurrence by age, breed and sex. Am J Vet Res 35:574, 1974.

3.   ACVO Genetics Committee, 1992 and/or Data from CERF All-Breeds Report, 1991.

MINIATURE SCHNAUZER

	DISORDER	INHERITANCE	REFERENCE	BREEDING ADVICE
A.	Congenital cataract and microphthalmia	Autosomal recessive	1	NO
B.	Cataract	Autosomal recessive	2	NO
C.	Progressive Retinal Atrophy	Autosomal recessive	3,4	NO

Description and Comments

A.   Congenital cataracts and microphthalmia

Congenital nuclear and posterior cortical lens opacities that progress slowly. In some cases, these cataracts appear similar to the congenital cataracts described in the following section (B). An associated abnormality in this defect is microphthalmia that is often mild and is accompanied by a 1-3 mm reduction in the axial length of the globe as determined by ultrasonography. Congenital cataracts and microphthalmia are inherited as an autosomal recessive disorder.

B.   Cataract

Lens opacity which may affect one or both eyes and may involve the lens partially or completely. In cases where cataracts are complete and affect both eyes, blindness results. The prudent approach is to assume cataracts to be hereditary except in cases known to be associated with trauma, other causes of ocular inflammation, specific metabolic diseases, persistent pupillary membranes, persistent hyaloid or nutritional deficiencies.

Congenital cataracts are bilateral and appear prior to 6 weeks of age. At this time they may already involve the entire lens. Others will first appear as posterior subcapsular opacities and usually progress to complete cataracts. These congenital cataracts are inherited as an autosomal recessive trait. There are other types of cataract in the breed which are potentially hereditary.

199

Note: It is not certain whether A and B are genetically distinct, or different manifestations of the same entity.

C.   Progressive Retinal Atrophy (PRA)

A degenerative disease of the retinal visual cells which progresses to blindness. This abnormality may be detected by electroretinogram before it is apparent clinically. In all breeds studied to date, PRA is recessively inherited.

In the miniature Schnauzer, PRA results from the abnormal development of visual cells followed by their slow degeneration. Although fundus abnormalities usually are not present until 3-5 years of age, abnormalities of the electroretinogram can be demonstrated by 8-10 weeks of age.

Other Conditions Under Consideration

D.   Low amplitude electroretinogram ("low amplitude")

This is a slowly progressive functional defect of the electroretinogram (ERG) that is characterized by a normal waveform but a lower than normal amplitude. "Low amplitude" has been detected as early as 16 weeks of age. When first detected, vision is normal and the retina is ophthalmoscopically normal. The significance of "low amplitude" is uncertain. Unpublished work (Parshall CJ and Aguirre G) suggests that animals having this functional deficit may develop PRA at a later age (10-13 years).

References

1.   Gelatt KN et al: Inheritance of congenital cataracts and microphthalmia in the miniature Schnauzer. Am J Vet Res 44: 1130, 1983.

2.   Rubin LF, Koch SA, Huber RJ: Hereditary cataracts in miniature Schnauzers. J Am Vet Med Assoc 154:1456, 1969.

3.   Aguirre G et al: Progressive retinal atrophy in the miniature Schnauzer. Trans Am Coll Vet Ophthalmol 16:226, 1985.

4.   Parshall C, Wyman M, Nitroy S, et al: Photoreceptor dysplasia: An inherited progressive retinal atrophy of miniature Schnauzer dogs. Prog Vet Comp Ophth 1:187, 1991.

NEAPOLITAN MASTIFF

	DISORDER	INHERITANCE	REFERENCE	BREEDING ADVICE
A.	Entropion	Not defined	1	Breeder option
B.	Ectropion / Macroblepharon	Not defined	1	Breeder option
C.	Dermoid	Not defined	1	Breeder option
D.	Eversion of cartilage of third eyelid	Not defined	1	Breeder option
E.	Prolapse of gland of third eyelid	Not defined	1	Breeder option
F.	Persistent pupillary membrane	Not defined	1	Breeder option
G.	Cataract	Not defined	1	NO
H.	Progressive Retinal Atrophy	Not defined	1	NO

Description and Comments

A.   Entropion

A conformational defect resulting in "in-rolling" of one or more of the eyelids which may cause ocular irritation. It is likely that entropion is influenced by several genes (polygenic), defining the skin and other structures which make up the eyelids, the amount and weight of the skin covering the head and face, the orbital contents and the conformation of the skull.

B.   Ectropion with Macroblepharon

Ectropion associated with an excessively large eyelid opening and laxity of the canthus structures. Central lower lid ectropion is often associated with entropion of the adjacent lid. This causes severe ocular irritation.

C.   Dermoid

A patch of skin, usually located on the cornea; its presence usually causes ocular irritation.

D.   Eversion of the cartilage of the third eyelid

A scroll-like curling of the cartilage of the third eyelid, usually everting the margin. The condition may occur in one or both eyes and may cause mild ocular irritation.

E.   Prolapse of the gland of the third eyelid

Protrusion of the tear gland associated with the third eyelid. The mode of inheritance of this disorder is unknown. The exposed gland may become irritated. Commonly referred to as "cherry eye".

F.   Persistent pupillary membranes (PPM)

Persistent blood vessel remnants in the anterior chamber of the eye which fail to regress normally in the neonatal period. These strands may bridge from iris to iris, iris to cornea, iris to lens, or form sheets of tissue in the anterior chamber. The last three forms pose the greatest threat to vision and when severe, vision impairment or blindness may occur.

G.   Cataract

Lens opacity which may affect one or both eyes and may involve the lens partially or completely. In cases where cataracts are complete and affect both eyes, blindness results. The prudent approach is to assume cataracts to be hereditary except in cases known to be associated with trauma, other causes of ocular inflammation, specific metabolic diseases, persistent pupillary membranes, persistent hyaloid or nutritional deficiencies.

H.   Progressive Retinal Atrophy (PRA)

A degenerative disease of the retinal visual cells which progresses to blindness. This abnormality may be detected by electroretinogram before it is apparent clinically. In all breeds studied to date, PRA is recessively inherited.

References

There are no references providing detailed descriptions of hereditary ocular conditions of the Neapolitan Mastiff breed. The conditions listed above are generally recognized to exist in this breed, as evidenced by repeated references made in general texts.

1.   ACVO Genetics Committee, 1992 and/or Data from CERF All-Breeds Report, 1991.

NEWFOUNDLAND

	DISORDER	INHERITANCE	REFERENCE	BREEDING ADVICE
A.	Ectropion	Not defined	1	Breeder option
B.	Macroblepharon	Not defined	1	Breeder option
C.	Entropion	Not defined	1	Breeder option
D.	Everted cartilage of third eyelid	Not defined	1	Breeder option
E.	Cataract	Not defined	1	NO

Description and Comments

A.   Ectropion

A conformational defect resulting in eversion of the eyelids, which may cause ocular irritation due to exposure. It is likely that ectropion is influenced by several genes (polygenic), defining the skin and other structures which make up the eyelids, the amount and weight of the skin covering the head and face, the orbital contents and the conformation of the skull.

B.   Macroblepharon

Abnormally large eyelid opening; may lead to secondary conditions associated with corneal exposure. In the Newfoundland, ectropion is associated with an exceptionally large palpebral fissure and laxity of the canthal structures. Central lower lid ectropion is often associated with entropion of the adjacent lid. This causes severe ocular irritation.

C.   Entropion

A conformational defect resulting in an "in-rolling" of one or more of the eyelids which may cause ocular irritation. It is likely that entropion is influenced by several genes (polygenic), defining the skin and other structures which make up the eyelids, the amount and weight of the skin covering the head and face, the orbital contents, and the conformation of the skull.

D.   Eversion of the cartilage of the third eyelid

A scroll-like curling of the cartilage of the third eyelid, usually everting the margin. The condition may occur in one or both eyes and may cause mild ocular irritation.

References

There are no references providing detailed descriptions of hereditary ocular conditions of the Newfoundland breed. The conditions listed above are generally recognized to exist in this breed, as evidenced by repeated references made in general texts.

1.   ACVO Genetics Committee, 1992 and/or Data from CERF All-Breeds Report, 1991.

NORWEGIAN ELKHOUND

	DISORDER	INHERITANCE	REFERENCE	BREEDING ADVICE
A.	Entropion	Not defined	1	Breeder option
B.	Glaucoma	Not defined	2,3	NO
C.	Lens luxation	Not defined	1	NO
D.	Progressive Retinal Atrophy			
	1. Rod dysplasia	Autosomal recessive	4-7	NO
	2. Early rod degeneration	Autosomal recessive	8,9	NO
E.	Cataract	Not defined	10	NO

Description and Comments

A.   Entropion

A conformational defect resulting in an "in-rolling" of one or more of the eyelids which may cause ocular irritation. It is likely that entropion is influenced by several genes (polygenic), defining the skin and other structures which make up the eyelids, the amount and weight of the skin covering the head and face, the orbital contents, and the conformation of the skull.

B.   Glaucoma

An elevation of intraocular pressure (IOP) which, when sustained, causes intraocular damage resulting in blindness. The elevated IOP occurs because the fluid cannot leave through the iridocorneal angle. Diagnosis and classification of glaucoma requires measurement of IOP (tonometry) and examination of the iridocorneal angle (gonioscopy). Neither of these tests are part of a routine breed eye screening exam.

Glaucoma may be secondary to lens luxation. However, some ophthalmologists feel this may be a distinct entity. The condition appears to be familial. In most cases the drainage angle is reported to be open.

C.   Lens luxation

Partial (subluxation) or complete displacement of the lens from the normal anatomic site behind the pupil. Lens luxation not associated with trauma or inflammation is presumed to be inherited. Lens luxation may result in elevated intraocular pressure (glaucoma) causing vision impairment or blindness.

Reported to have occurred in families of Elkhounds. The luxations occur from 2-6 years of age and are bilateral. Secondary glaucoma is common.

D.   Progressive Retinal Atrophy (PRA)

A degenerative disease of the retinal visual cells which progresses to blindness. This abnormality may be detected by electroretinogram before it is apparent clinically. In all breeds studied to date, PRA is recessively inherited.

1. Rod dysplasia: Inappropriate <u>development</u> of the visual cells resulting in vision impairment in dim light by 6 months and total blindness at 3-5 years. Ophthalmoscopic signs may be evident after 5 months of age, with signs of retinal vascular thinning after 2 years. An ERG can provide a diagnosis as early as 6 weeks of age. In the Elkhound, this is an autosomal recessive trait.

2. Early retinal degeneration: Another form of PRA reported in the Elkhound, animals are night blind at 6 weeks and blind by 1 year of age. Clinical signs are evident by 6 months. As with other forms of PRA, it is suspected to be an autosomal recessive disorder.

E.   Cataract

Lens opacity which may affect one or both eyes and may involve the lens partially or completely. In cases where cataracts are complete and affect both eyes, blindness results. The prudent approach is to assume cataracts to be hereditary except in cases known to be associated with trauma, other causes of ocular inflammation, specific metabolic diseases, persistent pupillary membranes, persistent hyaloid or nutritional deficiencies.

References

1.   Rubin LF: <u>Inherited Eye Diseases of Purebred Dogs</u>. Williams & Wilkins, 1989, p209.

2. Martin CL, Wyman M: Primary glaucoma in the dog. Vet Clin North Amer 8:257, 1978.

3. Slater MR, Erb HN: Effects of risk factors and prophylactic treatment on primary glaucoma in the dog. J Am Vet Med Assoc 188:1028, 1986.

4. Aguirre GD, Rubin LF: The early diagnosis of rod dysplasia in the Norwegian elkhound. J Am Vet Med Assoc 159:429, 1971.

5. Cogan DG, Kuwabara T: Photoreceptor abiotrophy of the retina in the elkhound. Path Vet 2:101, 1965.

6. Aguirre GD, Rubin LF: Progressive retinal atrophy (rod dysplasia) in the Norwegian elkhound. J Am Vet Med Assoc 158:208, 1970.

7. Aguirre GD, Rubin LF: An electrophysiologic approach for early diagnosis of progressive retinal atrophy in the Norwegian elkhound. J Am Anim Hosp Assoc 7:136, 1971.

8. Acland GM, Aguirre GD: Retinal degenerations in the dog: IV. Early retinal degeneration (erd) in Norwegian elkhounds. Exp Eye Res 44:491, 1987.

9. Acland GM, Aguirre GD, Parkes J, Liebman P: A new early onset inherited retinal degeneration in the Norwegian elkhound. Trans Am Coll Vet Ophthalmol 1983, 98.

10. ACVO Genetics Committee, 1992 and/or Data from CERF All-Breeds Report, 1991.

NOVA SCOTIA DUCK TOLLING RETRIEVER

	DISORDER	INHERITANCE	REFERENCE	BREEDING ADVICE
A.	Progressive Retinal Atrophy	Not defined	1,2	NO
B.	Cataract	Not defined	2	NO

Description and Comments

A.   Progressive Retinal Atrophy (PRA)

A degenerative disease of the retinal visual cells which progresses to blindness. This abnormality may be detected by electroretinogram before it is apparent clinically. In all breeds studied to date, PRA is recessively inherited. In this breed, inheritance appears to be autosomal recessive. Clinical onset is reported at 5-6 years of age.

B.   Cataract

Lens opacity which may affect one or both eyes and may involve the lens partially or completely. In cases where cataracts are complete and affect both eyes, blindness results. The prudent approach is to assume cataracts to be hereditary except in cases known to be associated with trauma, other causes of ocular inflammation, specific metabolic diseases, persistent pupillary membranes, persistent hyaloid or nutritional deficiencies. Cataract may be seen in association with PRA.

References

There are no references providing detailed descriptions of hereditary ocular conditions of the Nova Scotia Duck Tolling Retriever breed. The conditions listed above are generally recognized to exist in this breed, as evidenced by repeated references made in general texts.

1.   ACVO Genetics Committee, 1992 and/or Data from CERF All-Breeds Report, 1991.

2.   Nova Scotia Duck Tolling Retriever Club of Canada, December 1990.

OLD ENGLISH SHEEPDOG

	DISORDER	INHERITANCE	REFERENCE	BREEDING ADVICE
A.	Distichiasis	Not defined	1,2	Breeder option
B.	Entropion	Not defined	3	Breeder option
C.	Cataract	Not defined	2,4	NO
D.	Progressive Retinal Atrophy	Not defined	3	NO
E.	Microphthalmia/ Multiple anomalies	Not defined	3	NO
F.	Retinal detachment	Not defined	4	NO

Description and Comments

A. Distichiasis

Eyelashes abnormally located in the eyelid margin which may cause ocular irritation. Distichiasis may occur at any time in the life of a dog. It is difficult to make a strong recommendation with regard to breeding dogs with this entity. The hereditary basis has not been established although it seems probable due to the high incidence in some breeds. Reducing the incidence is a logical goal. When diagnosed, distichiasis should be recorded; breeding discretion is advised.

B. Entropion

A conformational defect resulting in an "in-rolling" of one or more of the eyelids which may cause ocular irritation. It is likely that entropion is influenced by several genes (polygenic), defining the skin and other structures which make up the eyelids, the amount and weight of the skin covering the head and face, the orbital contents, and the conformation of the skull.

C. Cataract

Lens opacity which may affect one or both eyes and may involve the lens partially or completely. In cases where cataracts are complete and affect both eyes, blindness results. The prudent approach is to assume cataracts to be hereditary except in cases known to be associated with trauma, other causes of ocular inflammation, specific metabolic diseases, persistent pupillary membranes, persistent hyaloid or nutritional deficiencies.

In the Old English Sheepdog, cataract may be seen with retinal detachment.

D. Progressive Retinal Atrophy (PRA)

A degenerative disease of the retinal visual cells which progresses to blindness. This abnormality may be detected by electroretinogram before it is apparent clinically. In all breeds studied to date, PRA is recessively inherited.

E. Microphthalmia and multiple congenital ocular defects

Microphthalmia is a developmental anomaly in which the eyeball is abnormally small. This is often associated with other ocular malformations, including defects of the cornea, anterior chamber, lens and/or retina.

Microphthalmia with cataract and retinal abnormalities has been reported in litters of Old English Sheepdogs. Lesions were non-progressive. However, blindness did result in some dogs. The mode of inheritance is unknown, but affected dogs should not be bred.

F. Retinal detachment

The separation of the sensory retina from the underlying tissue. It results in blindness when complete. In the OES, retinal detachment has been seen with cataracts. The relationship between the two conditions is not defined.

Other Conditions Under Consideration

G. Corneal dystrophy

A non-inflammatory corneal opacity (white to gray) present in one or more of the corneal layers; usually inherited and bilateral. In the OES, dystrophy of the corneal endothelium has been reported.

H.   Sclero-uveitis

An inflammatory disease of the sclera and uvea; the condition may be serious enough to cause blindness.

References

1.   Barnett KC: Comparative aspects of canine hereditary disease. Adv Vet Sci Comp Med 20:39, 1976.

2.   Smythe RH: <u>Veterinary Ophthalmology</u>, ed.2, London, Balliere Tindall and Cox, 1958.

3.   Rubin LF: <u>Inherited Eye Diseases in Purebred Dogs</u>. Williams & Wilkins, 1989, p214.

4.   Koch SA: Cataracts in interrelated Old English sheepdogs. J Am Vet Med Assoc 160:299, 1972.

PAPILLON

	DISORDER	INHERITANCE	REFERENCE	BREEDING ADVICE
A.	Entropion	Not defined	1,2	Breeder option
B.	Cataract	Not defined	1,2	NO
C.	Corneal dystrophy	Not defined	1	Breeder option

Description and Comments

A.   Entropion

A conformational defect resulting in an "in-rolling" of one or more of the eyelids which may cause ocular irritation. It is likely that entropion is influenced by several genes (polygenic), defining the skin and other structures which make up the eyelids, the amount and weight of the skin covering the head and face, the orbital contents, and the conformation of the skull. In the Papillon, entropion usually involves the medial canthal margin of the lower eyelid(s).

B.   Cataract

Lens opacity which may affect one or both eyes and may involve the lens partially or completely. In cases where cataracts are complete and affect both eyes, blindness results. The prudent approach is to assume cataracts to be hereditary except in cases known to be associated with trauma, other causes of ocular inflammation, specific metabolic diseases, persistent pupillary membranes, persistent hyaloid or nutritional deficiencies. Nuclear and posterior cortical cataracts have been reported in the Papillon.

C.   Corneal dystrophy

A non-inflammatory corneal opacity (white to gray) present in one or more of the corneal layers; usually inherited and bilateral.

References

There are no references providing detailed descriptions of hereditary ocular conditions of the Papillon breed. The conditions listed above are generally recognized to exist in this breed, as evidenced by repeated references made in general texts.

1.   ACVO Genetics Committee, 1992 and/or Data from CERF All-Breeds Report, 1991.

2.   Rubin LF: Inherited Eye Diseases in Purebred Dogs. Williams & Wilkins, Baltimore, 1989, p218.

PEKINGESE

	DISORDER	INHERITANCE	REFERENCE	BREEDING ADVICE
A.	Distichiasis	Not defined	1,4	Breeder option
B.	Entropion	Not defined	3	Breeder option
C.	Exposure keratopathy syndrome	Not defined	3	NO
D.	Progressive Retinal Atrophy	Not defined	2,3	NO
E.	Cataract	Not defined	5	NO
F.	Dry Eye	Not defined	5	NO
G.	Ciliated caruncle	Not defined	5	Breeder option

Description and Comments

A.   Distichiasis

Eyelashes abnormally located in the eyelid margin which may cause ocular irritation. Distichiasis may occur at any time in the life of a dog. It is difficult to make a strong recommendation with regard to breeding dogs with this entity. The hereditary basis has not been established although it seems probable due to the high incidence in some breeds. Reducing the incidence is a logical goal. When diagnosed, distichiasis should be recorded; breeding discretion is advised.

B.   Entropion

A conformational defect resulting in an "in-rolling" of one or more of the eyelids which may cause ocular irritation. It is likely that entropion is influenced by several genes (polygenic), defining the skin and other structures which make up the eyelids, the amount and weight of the skin covering the head and face, the orbital contents, and the conformation of the skull.

C.   Exposure keratopathy syndrome

A corneal disease involving all or part of the cornea, resulting from inadequate blinking. This results from a combination of anatomic features including shallow orbits, exophthalmos, macroblepharon and lagophthalmos.

D.   Progressive Retinal Atrophy (PRA)

A degenerative disease of the retinal visual cells which progresses to blindness. This abnormality may be detected by electroretinogram before it is apparent clinically. In all breeds studied to date, PRA is recessively inherited.

E.   Cataract

Lens opacity which may affect one or both eyes and may involve the lens partially or completely. In cases where cataracts are complete and affect both eyes, blindness results. The prudent approach is to assume cataracts to be hereditary except in cases known to be associated with trauma, other causes of ocular inflammation, specific metabolic diseases, persistent pupillary membranes, persistent hyaloid or nutritional deficiencies.

F.   Dry eye

An abnormality of the tear film, most commonly a deficiency of the aqueous portion, although the mucin and/or lipid layers may be affected; results in ocular irritation and/or vision impairment.

G.   Ciliated caruncle

Fleshy conjunctival tissue at the nasal canthus; may contain hair (ciliated caruncle) which, if contacting the cornea, may cause irritation and/or tearing.

References

1.   Barnett KC: Comparative aspects of canine hereditary eye disease. Adv Vet Sci Comp Med 20:39, 1976.

2.   Priester WA: Canine progressive retinal atrophy: Occurrence by age, breed and sex. Am J Vet Res 35:571, 1974.

3.   Whitley RD, Miller TR: Predisposition to ocular disease in dogs. Proc CAVO and ASVO Joint Meeting in conjunction with the 23rd World Veterinary Congress, 1987, p20.

4. Gelatt KN: Pediatric ophthalmology in small animal practice. Vet Clin North Amer 3:321,1973.

5. ACVO Genetics Committee, 1992 and/or Data from CERF All-Breeds Report, 1991.

POINTER

	DISORDER	INHERITANCE	REFERENCE	BREEDING ADVICE
A.	Entropion	Not defined	1	Breeder option
B.	Cataract	Not defined	2,3	NO
C.	Progressive Retinal Atrophy	Not defined	4,5	NO

Description and Comments

A.   Entropion

A conformational defect resulting in "in-rolling" of one or more of the eyelids which may cause ocular irritation. It is likely that entropion is influenced by several genes (polygenic), defining the skin and other structures which make up the eyelids, the amount and weight of the skin covering the head and face, the orbital contents and the conformation of the skull.

B.   Cataract

Lens opacity which may affect one or both eyes and may involve the lens partially or completely. In cases where cataracts are complete and affect both eyes, blindness results. The prudent approach is to assume cataracts to be hereditary except in cases known to be associated with trauma, other causes of ocular inflammation, specific metabolic diseases, persistent pupillary membranes, persistent hyaloid or nutritional deficiencies. Onset in the Pointer is 2-3 years of age. Opacities occur at the lens periphery and progress to impair vision. May be seen with PRA.

C.   Progressive Retinal Atrophy (PRA)

A degenerative disease of the retinal visual cells which progresses to blindness. This abnormality may be detected by electroretinogram before it is apparent clinically. In all breeds studied to date, PRA is recessively inherited. Clinical onset in the Pointer is 5-6 years of age.

218

Other Conditions Under Consideration

D.   Corneal dystrophy

A non-inflammatory corneal opacity (white to gray) present in one or more of the corneal layers; usually inherited and bilateral. A lipid dystrophy resembling that reported in the Siberian Husky has been seen in Pointers 6 years old.

E.   Pannus / Chronic Superficial Keratitis

A bilateral disease of the cornea which usually starts as a grayish haze to the ventral or ventrolateral cornea, followed by the formation of a vascularized subepithelial growth that begins to spread toward the central cornea; pigmentation follows the vascularization. If severe, vision impairment occurs.

References

There are no references providing detailed descriptions of hereditary ocular conditions of the Pointer breed. The conditions listed above are generally recognized to exist in this breed, as evidenced by repeated references made in general texts.

1.   Burns M, Fraser MN: Genetics of the dog, ed 2. Edinburgh, Oliver and Boyd, 1966.

2.   Host P, Sveinson S: Arselig katarakt hos hunder (Inherited cataract in dogs). Norsk Vet Tidskr 48:244, 1936.

3.   Rubin, LF: Inherited Eye Diseases in Purebred Dogs. Williams and Wilkins, Baltimore, 1989.

4.   Magrane WG: Canine Ophthalmology, ed 3. Philadelphia, Lea and Febiger, 1977.

5.   Priester WA: Canine progressive retinal atrophy. Occurrence by age, breed and sex. Am J Vet Res 35:571, 1974.

POMERANIAN

	DISORDER	INHERITANCE	REFERENCE	BREEDING ADVICE
A.	Entropion	Not defined	1,2	Breeder option
B.	Cataract	Not defined	3	NO
C.	Progressive Retinal Atrophy	Not defined	3	NO

Description and Comments

A. Entropion

A conformational defect resulting in an "in-rolling" of one or more of the eyelids which may cause ocular irritation. It is likely that entropion is influenced by several genes (polygenic), defining the skin and other structures which make up the eyelids, the amount and weight of the skin covering the head and face, the orbital contents, and the conformation of the skull. In the Pomeranian, entropion usually involves the medial canthal margin of the lower eyelid(s).

B. Cataract

Lens opacity which may affect one or both eyes and may involve the lens partially or completely. In cases where cataracts are complete and affect both eyes, blindness results. The prudent approach is to assume cataracts to be hereditary except in cases known to be associated with trauma, other causes of ocular inflammation, specific metabolic diseases, persistent pupillary membranes, persistent hyaloid or nutritional deficiencies.

C. Progressive Retinal Atrophy (PRA)

A degenerative disease of the retinal visual cells which progresses to blindness. This abnormality may be detected by electroretinogram before it is apparent clinically. In all breeds studied to date, PRA is recessively inherited.

References

There are no references providing detailed descriptions of hereditary ocular conditions of the Pomeranian breed. The conditions listed above are generally recognized to exist in this breed, as evidenced by repeated references made in general texts.

1.   Barnett KC: Comparative aspects of canine hereditary eye disease. Adv Sci Comp Med 20:39, 1976.

2.   Gray H: The diseases of the eye in domesticated animals. Vet Rec 21:678, 1909.

3.   Rubin LF: <u>Inherited Eye Diseases in Purebred Dogs</u>. Williams & Wilkins, 1989, p226.

POODLE
(Toy, Miniature, and Standard)

All varieties of the Poodle are basically the same genetic makeup, having their size governed by differences in an "insulin-like growth factor". (See Reference 1)

	DISORDER	INHERITANCE	REFERENCE	BREEDING ADVICE
A.	Progressive Retinal Atrophy	Autosomal recessive	2-8	NO
B.	Micropapilla	Not defined	9	NO
C.	Cataract	Not defined	10	NO
D.	Microphthalmia	Not defined	--	NO
E.	Glaucoma	Not defined	--	NO
F.	Entropion	Not defined	--	NO
G.	Imperforate lacrimal puncta	Not defined	--	Breeder option
H.	Distichiasis	Not defined	--	Breeder option

Description and Comments

A.   Progressive Retinal Atrophy (PRA)

A degenerative disease of the retinal visual cells which progresses to blindness. This abnormality may be detected by electroretinogram before it is apparent clinically. In all breeds studied to date, PRA is recessively inherited.

Progressive rod/cone degeneration is the term used for the entity described as PRA in the poodle. It may be detected ophthalmoscopically as early as 3 years of age; however, some animals may be detected earlier. Diagnostic electroretinography (ERG) is usually required in younger animals to detect signs of retinal rod/cone cell failure <u>before</u> signs can be seen ophthalmoscopically. The mode of inheritance is considered to be an autosomal recessive trait.

B.   Micropapilla

A small optic disc which is not associated with vision impairment. May be unable to differentiate from optic nerve hypoplasia on a routine (dilated) screening ophthalmoscopic exam.

Hypoplastic optic nerve is a condition of failure of the complete development of the optic nerve. The signs have a variety of expression and degrees of hypoplasia can be found. One or both eyes may be affected. Affected eyes may retain some function or be blind. The mode of inheritance is not clear.

C.   Cataract

Lens opacity which may affect one or both eyes and may involve the lens partially or completely. In cases where cataracts are complete and affect both eyes, blindness results. The prudent approach is to assume cataracts to be hereditary except in cases known to be associated with trauma, other causes of ocular inflammation, specific metabolic diseases, persistent pupillary membranes, persistent hyaloid or nutritional deficiencies.

The poodle cataract can involve the lens cortex and lens nucleus. The rate and degree of progression are variable. A familial form of cataract has been described in the standard poodle, progressing from an equatorial opacity.

D.   Microphthalmia / multiple congenital ocular defects

Microphthalmia is a developmental anomaly in which the eyeball is abnormally small. This is often associated with other ocular malformations, including defects in the cornea, anterior chamber, lens and/or retina. It can be found in one or both eyes. The mode of inheritance is not known.

E.   Glaucoma

An elevation of intraocular pressure (IOP) which, when sustained, causes intraocular damage resulting in blindness. The elevated IOP occurs because the fluid cannot leave through the iridocorneal angle. Diagnosis and classification of glaucoma requires measurement of IOP (tonometry) and examination of the iridocorneal angle (gonioscopy). Neither of these tests are part of a routine breed eye screening exam.

The poodle form is usually a narrow angle variety and often associated with a condition of goniodysgenesis (a condition of incomplete formation and development of the iridocorneal angle).

F.   Entropion

A conformational defect resulting in an "in-rolling" of one or more of the eyelids which may cause ocular irritation. It is likely that entropion is influenced by several genes (polygenic), defining the skin and other structures which make up the eyelids, the amount and weight of the skin covering the head and face, the orbital contents, and the conformation of the skull. Selection should be directed against entropion and toward a head conformation that minimizes or eliminates the likelihood of the defect.

G.   Imperforate lacrimal punctum

A developmental abnormality resulting in failure of opening of the lacrimal duct adjacent to the eye. The lower punctum is more frequently affected. This defect usually results in epiphora, a overflow of tears onto the face.

H.   Distichiasis

Eyelashes abnormally located in the eyelid margin which may cause ocular irritation. Distichiasis may occur at any time in the life of a dog. It is difficult to make a strong recommendation with regard to breeding dogs with this entity. The hereditary basis has not been established although it seems probable due to the high incidence in some breeds. Reducing the incidence is a logical goal. When diagnosed, distichiasis should be recorded; breeding discretion is advised.

Other Conditions Under Consideration

I.   Ectopic cilia

Hair emerging through the eyelid conjunctiva. Ectopic cilia occur more frequently in younger dogs and cause discomfort and corneal disease.

References

1.   Eigenmann JE et al: Body size parallels insulin-like growth factor I levels but not growth hormone secretory capacity. ACTA Endocrinol 106:448, 1984.

2.   Aguirre GD: Inherited retinal degeneration in the dog. Trans Acad Ophth Otol 81:667, 1976.

3.   Aguirre GD, Rubin LF: Progressive retinal atrophy in the miniature poodle: an electrophysiologic study. J Am Vet Med Assoc 160:191, 1972.

4. American College of Veterinary Ophthalmologists: Committee on progressive retinal atrophy, Parshall et al: Summary report, 1976.

5. Aguirre GD et al: Hereditary retinal degeneration in the dog: Specificity of abnormal cyclic nucleotide metabolism to diseases of arrested photoreceptor development. Birth Defects 18:119, 1982.

6. Aguirre GD et al: Pathogenesis of progressive rod-cone degeneration in miniature poodles. Invest Ophthalmol Vis Sci 23:610, 1982.

7. Parkes J et al: Progressive rod-cone degeneration in the dog: Characterization of the visual pigment. Invest Ophthalmol Vis Sci 23:674, 1982.

8. Aguirre G, O'Brien P: Morphological and biochemical studies of canine progressive rod-cone degeneration. Invest Ophthalmol Vis Sci 27:635, 1986.

9. Kern TJ, Riis RC: Optic nerve hypoplasia in three miniature poodles. J Am Vet Med Assoc 178:49, 1981.

10. Rubin LF, Flowers RD: Inherited cataract in a family of standard poodles. J Am Vet Med Assoc 161:207, 1972.

PORTUGUESE WATER DOG

	DISORDER	INHERITANCE	REFERENCE	BREEDING ADVICE
A.	Microphthalmia and multiple congenital ocular anomalies	Not defined	1	NO
B.	Distichiasis	Not defined	2	Breeder option
C.	Cataracts	Not defined	--	NO
D.	Persistent pupillary membranes	Not defined	--	Breeder option
E.	Progressive Retinal Atrophy	Not defined	2	NO

Description and Comments

A.   Microphthalmia and multiple congenital ocular anomalies

This is a congenital abnormality present bilaterally and characterized by a small globe and associated ocular defects which can affect the cornea, anterior chamber, lens and/or retina. These associated defects may be variable in severity. Several cases have been identified, all of which appeared to have a common ancestry. All affected animals so far identified have been the progeny of dogs that were phenotypically normal, suggesting that the defect is not dominantly inherited.

B.   Distichiasis

Eyelashes abnormally located in the eyelid margin which may cause ocular irritation. Distichiasis may occur at any time in the life of a dog. It is difficult to make a strong recommendation with regard to breeding dogs with this entity. The hereditary basis has not been established, although it seems probable due to the high incidence in some breeds. Reducing the incidence is a logical goal. When diagnosed, distichiasis should be recorded; breeding discretion is advised.

C. Cataracts

Lens opacity which may affect one or both eyes and may involve the lens partially or completely. In cases where cataracts are complete and affect both eyes, blindness results. The prudent approach is to assume cataracts to be hereditary except in cases known to be associated with trauma, other causes of ocular inflammation, specific metabolic diseases, persistent pupillary membranes, persistent hyaloid or nutritional deficiencies. The exact frequency and significance of cataracts in the breed is not known.

D. Persistent pupillary membranes

Persistent blood vessel remnants in the anterior chamber of the eye which fail to regress normally in the neonatal period. These strands may bridge from iris to iris, iris to cornea, iris to lens, or form sheets of tissue in the anterior chamber. The last three forms pose the greatest threat to vision and when severe, vision impairment or blindness may occur. The exact frequency and significance of this disorder in the breed is not known.

E. Progressive Retinal Atrophy (PRA)

A degenerative disease of the retinal visual cells which progresses to blindness. This abnormality may be detected by electroretinogram before it is apparent clinically. In all breeds studied to date, PRA is recessively inherited.

The disease in the Portuguese Water Dog has not been characterized sufficiently to establish a disease frequency, the disease mechanism, or the age when early diagnosis by ophthalmoscopy and/or electroretinography is possible. In most affected dogs to date, the disease is recognized clinically in dogs 3-5 years of age or older; this suggests that the disease represents one of the late-onset forms of PRA.

References

1. Case records (1986-present), Section of Medical Genetics, School of Veterinary Medicine, University of Pennsylvania.

2. ACVO Genetics Committee, 1992 and/or Data from CERF All-Breeds Report, 1991.

PUG

	DISORDER	INHERITANCE	REFERENCE	BREEDING ADVICE
A.	Distichiasis	Not defined	1,2	Breeder option
B.	Entropion	Not defined	1,2	Breeder option
C.	Exposure keratopathy syndrome	Polygenic	1,3,4,5	Breeder option

Description and Comments

A. Distichiasis

Eyelashes abnormally located in the eyelid margin which may cause ocular irritation. Distichiasis may occur at any time in the life of a dog. It is difficult to make a strong recommendation with regard to breeding dogs with this entity. The hereditary basis has not been established although it seems probable due to the high incidence in some breeds. Reducing the incidence is a logical goal. When diagnosed, distichiasis should be recorded; breeding discretion is advised.

B. Entropion

A conformational defect resulting in an "in-rolling" of one or more of the eyelids which may cause ocular irritation. It is likely that entropion is influenced by several genes (polygenic), defining the skin and other structures which make up the eyelids, the amount and weight of the skin covering the head and face, the orbital contents, and the conformation of the skull. In the Pug, entropion usually involves the medial canthal margin of the lower eyelid(s).

C. Exposure keratopathy syndrome

A corneal disease involving all or part of the cornea, resulting from inadequate blinking. This results from a combination of anatomic features including shallow orbits, exophthalmos, macroblepharon and lagophthalmos. The breed standard indicates the Pug should have a "large massive round head with very large, bold and prominent eyes". These characteristics give rise to the ocular exposure and irritative problems common in the breed.

Other Conditions Under Consideration

D.   Cataract

Lens opacity which may affect one or both eyes and may involve the lens partially or completely. In cases where cataracts are complete and affect both eyes, blindness results. The prudent approach is to assume cataracts to be hereditary except in cases known to be associated with trauma, other causes of ocular inflammation, specific metabolic diseases, persistent pupillary membranes, persistent hyaloid or nutritional deficiencies.

References

There are no references providing detailed descriptions of hereditary ocular conditions of the Pug breed. The conditions listed above are generally recognized to exist in this breed, as evidenced by repeated references made in general texts.

1.   ACVO Genetics Committee, 1992 and/or Data from CERF All-Breeds Report, 1991.

2.   Rubin LF: Inherited Eye Diseases in Purebred Dogs. Williams and Wilkins, Baltimore, 1989, p241.

3.   Wyman M: Manual of Small Animal Ophthalmology. Churchill Livingstone, New York, 1986.

4.   American Kennel Club: The Complete Dog Book, ed 17, Howell Book House Inc, New York, 1985.

5.   Hodgman SFJ: Abnormalities and defects in pedigree dogs I. An investigation into the existence of abnormalities in pedigree dogs in the British Isles. J Small Anim Pract 4: 447, 1963.

PULI

	DISORDER	INHERITANCE	REFERENCE	BREEDING ADVICE
A.	Cataract	Not defined	--	NO
B.	Progressive Retinal Atrophy	Not defined	--	NO
C.	Retinal dysplasia - folds	Not defined	--	Breeder option

Description and Comments

A.   Cataract

Lens opacity which may affect one or both eyes and may involve the lens partially or completely. In cases where cataracts are complete and affect both eyes, blindness results. The prudent approach is to assume cataracts to be hereditary except in cases known to be associated with trauma, other causes of ocular inflammation, specific metabolic diseases, persistent pupillary membranes, persistent hyaloid or nutritional deficiencies.

B.   Progressive Retinal Atrophy

A degenerative disease of the retinal visual cells which progresses to blindness. This abnormality may be detected by electroretinogram before it is apparent clinically. In all breeds studied to date, PRA is recessively inherited.

C.   Retinal dysplasia

Abnormal development of the retina present at birth and recognized to have three forms:

1) Retinal dysplasia - **folds**: linear, triangular, curved or curvilinear foci of retinal folding that may be single or multiple.
2) Retinal dysplasia - **geographic**: any irregularly shaped area of abnormal retinal development, representing changes not accountable by simple folding.

3) Retinal dysplasia - **detachment**: either of the above described forms of retinal dysplasia associated with separation (detachment) of the retina.

The two latter forms are associated with vision impairment or blindness. Retinal dysplasia is known to be inherited in many breeds. The genetic relationship between the three forms of the disease is not known for all breeds.

References

There are no references providing detailed descriptions of hereditary ocular conditions of the Puli breed. The conditions listed above are generally recognized to exist in this breed, as evidenced by repeated references made in general texts.

1. ACVO Genetics Committee, 1992 and/or Data from CERF All-Breeds Report, 1991.

REDBONE HOUND

DISORDER	INHERITANCE	REFERENCE	BREEDING ADVICE
A. Entropion	Not defined	1	NO
B. Ectropion	Not defined	1	Breeder option

Description and Comments

A. Entropion

A conformational defect resulting in "in-rolling" of one or more of the eyelids which may cause ocular irritation. It is likely that entropion is influenced by several genes (polygenic), defining the skin and other structures which make up the eyelids, the amount and weight of the skin covering the head and face, the orbital contents and the conformation of the skull

B. Ectropion

A conformational defect resulting in eversion of the eyelids, which may cause ocular irritation due to exposure. It is likely that ectropion is influenced by several genes (polygenic), defining the skin and other structures which make up the eyelids, the amount and weight of the skin covering the head and face, the orbital contents and the conformation of the skull.

References

There are no references providing detailed descriptions of hereditary ocular conditions of the Red Bone Hound breed. The conditions listed above are generally recognized to exist in this breed, as evidenced by repeated references made in general texts.

1. ACVO Genetics Committee, 1992 and/or Data from CERF All-Breeds Report, 1991.

RHODESIAN RIDGEBACK

	DISORDER	INHERITANCE	REFERENCE	BREEDING ADVICE
A.	Entropion	Not defined	1	Breeder option
B.	Progressive Retinal Atrophy	Not defined	1	NO

Description and Comments

A.   Entropion

A conformational defect resulting in "in-rolling" of one or more of the eyelids which may cause ocular irritation. It is likely that entropion is influenced by several genes (polygenic), defining the skin and other structures which make up the eyelids, the amount and weight of the skin covering the head and face, the orbital contents and the conformation of the skull.

B.   Progressive Retinal Atrophy (PRA)

A degenerative disease of the retinal visual cells which progresses to blindness. This abnormality may be detected by electroretinogram before it is apparent clinically. In all breeds studied to date, PRA is recessively inherited.

References

There are no references providing detailed descriptions of hereditary ocular conditions of the Rhodesian Ridgeback breed. The conditions listed above are generally recognized to exist in this breed, as evidenced by repeated references made in general texts.

1.   ACVO Genetics Committee, 1992 and/or Data from CERF All-Breeds Report, 1991.

ROTTWEILER

	DISORDER	INHERITANCE	REFERENCE	BREEDING ADVICE
A.	Entropion	Not defined	1	Breeder option
B.	Distichiasis	Not defined	1	Breeder option
C.	Cataract	Not defined	1	NO
D.	Progressive Retinal Atrophy	Not defined	1	NO
E.	Iris coloboma	Not defined	1	NO
F.	Retinal dysplasia	Not defined	1	Breeder option

Description and Comments

A.   Entropion

A conformational defect resulting in an "in-rolling" of one or more of the eyelids which may cause ocular irritation. It is likely that entropion is influenced by several genes (polygenic), defining the skin and other structures which make up the eyelids, the amount and weight of the skin covering the head and face, the orbital contents, and the conformation of the skull.

Entropion in the Rottweiler has been observed with increasing frequency in the past few years. Selection should be directed against entropion and toward a head conformation that minimizes or eliminates the likelihood of the defect. The entropion usually involves the lower eyelids in this breed and requires surgical correction.

B.   Distichiasis

Eyelashes abnormally located in the eyelid margin which may cause ocular irritation. Distichiasis may occur at any time in the life of a dog. It is difficult to make a strong recommendation with regard to breeding dogs with this entity. The hereditary basis has not been established although it seems probable due to the high incidence in some breeds. Reducing the incidence is a logical goal. When diagnosed, distichiasis should be recorded. Breeding discretion is advised.

C. Cataract

Lens opacity which may affect one or both eyes and may involve the lens partially or completely. In cases where cataracts are complete and affect both eyes, blindness results. The prudent approach is to assume cataracts to be hereditary except in cases known to be associated with trauma, other causes of ocular inflammation, specific metabolic diseases, persistent pupillary membranes, persistent hyaloid or nutritional deficiencies.

A variety of cataracts have been observed in this breed ranging from the posterior polar cataract similar to that in the Golden retriever and cataracts involving multiple areas of the nucleus and cortex. Further studies need to be performed as to the exact cause, but it is our recommendation that the individually afflicted dog should not be bred.

D. Progressive Retinal Atrophy (PRA)

A degenerative disease of the retinal visual cells which progresses to blindness. This abnormality may be detected by electroretinogram before it is apparent clinically. In all breeds studied to date, PRA is recessively inherited.

A tapetal color change has been noted in the Rottweiler that may or may not progress. Its relationship (if any) to PRA is unknown.

E. Iris coloboma

A developmental anomaly in which a portion of the iris is absent. It may be a separate disorder or associated with other ocular malformations.

A few Rottweilers have been observed with a congenital iris defect in the nasal half in which large areas of iris tissue are missing bilaterally. This does not appear to be a progressive disease but there have been patients observed with the entire nasal half of the iris involved.

F. Retinal dysplasia

Abnormal development of the retina present at birth and recognized to have three forms:

1) Retinal dysplasia - **folds**: linear, triangular, curved or curvilinear foci of retinal folding that may be single or multiple.

2) Retinal dysplasia - **geographic**: any irregularly shaped area of abnormal retinal development, representing changes not accountable by simple folding.

3) Retinal dysplasia - **detachment**: either of the above described forms of retinal dysplasia associated with separation (detachment) of the retina.

The two latter forms are associated with vision impairment or blindness. Retinal dysplasia is known to be inherited in many breeds. The genetic relationship between the three forms of the disease is not known for all breeds.

The Rottweiler retinal dysplasia takes the form of focal abnormal development and to date no visual impairment has been observed. The condition does not appear to be progressive.

References

There are no references providing detailed descriptions of hereditary ocular conditions of the Rottweiler breed. The conditions listed above are generally recognized to exist in this breed, as evidenced by repeated references made in general texts.

1.   ACVO Genetics Committee, 1992 and/or Data from CERF All-Breeds Report, 1991.

SAINT BERNARD

	DISORDER	INHERITANCE	REFERENCE	BREEDING ADVICE
A.	Entropion	Not defined	1	NO
B.	Ectropion	Not defined	--	Breeder option
C.	Distichiasis	Not defined	2	Breeder option
D.	Dermoid	Not defined	2-4	Breeder option
E.	Cataract	Not defined	--	NO
F.	Multiple ocular defects	Not defined	5	NO

Description and Comments

A.   Entropion

A conformational defect resulting in an "in-rolling" of one or more of the eyelids which may cause ocular irritation. It is likely that entropion is influenced by several genes (polygenic), defining the skin and other structures which make up the eyelids, the amount and weight of the skin covering the head and face, the orbital contents, and the conformation of the skull. In this breed, entropion is associated with an exceptionally large palpebral fissure.

B.   Ectropion

A conformational defect resulting in eversion of the eyelids which may cause ocular irritation. It is likely that ectropion is influenced by several genes (polygenic) defining the skin and other structures which make up the eyelids, the amount and weight of the skin covering the head and face, the orbital contents and the conformation of the skull.

C.   Distichiasis

Eyelashes abnormally located in the eyelid margin which may cause ocular irritation. Distichiasis may occur at any time in the life of a dog. It is difficult to make a strong recommendation with regard to breeding dogs with this entity. The hereditary basis has not been established although it seems probable due to the high incidence in some breeds. Reducing the incidence is a logical goal. When diagnosed, distichiasis should be recorded; breeding discretion is advised.

D.   Dermoid

A patch of skin, usually located on the cornea; its presence usually causes ocular irritation.

E.   Cataract

Lens opacity which may affect one or both eyes and may involve the lens partially or completely. In cases where cataracts are complete and affect both eyes, blindness results. The prudent approach is to assume cataracts to be hereditary except in cases known to be associated with trauma, other causes of ocular inflammation, specific metabolic diseases, persistent pupillary membranes, persistent hyaloid or nutritional deficiencies.

F.   Multiple ocular defects

Multiple ocular defects have been described in Saint Bernard puppies. The syndrome was composed of microphthalmia, microphakia, aphakia, acorea, peripheral anterior synechia, and retinal dysplasia. Glaucoma was also reported. Although the cause was not proven to be hereditary, the fact that several of these dogs were related suggests a hereditary basis. Affected dogs should not be bred.

References

1.   Hodgman SFJ: Abnormalities and defects in pedigree dogs I. An investigation into the existence of abnormalities in pedigree dogs in the British Isles. J Small Anim Pract 4:447, 1963.

2.   Gelatt KN: Bilateral corneal dermoids and distichiasis in a dog. Vet Med 66:658, 1971.

3.   Kittel H: Deut Tieraerztl Wochenschr 52:793, 1931.

4. Burns M, Fraser MN. <u>Genetics of the Dog</u>. Oliver and Boyd, Edinburgh and London, 1966.

5. Martin CL, Leipold HW: Aphakia and multiple ocular defects in Saint Bernard puppies. Vet Med Small Anim Clin 69:448, 1974.

SALUKI

DISORDER	INHERITANCE	REFERENCE	BREEDING ADVICE
A. Cataract	Not defined	--	NO

Description and Comments

A.   Cataract

Lens opacity which may affect one or both eyes and may involve the lens partially or completely. In cases where cataracts are complete and affect both eyes, blindness results. The prudent approach is to assume cataracts to be hereditary except in cases known to be associated with trauma, other causes of ocular inflammation, specific metabolic diseases, persistent pupillary membranes, persistent hyaloid or nutritional deficiencies.

Other Conditions Under Consideration

B.   Entropion

A conformational defect resulting in an "in-rolling" of one or more of the eyelids which may cause ocular irritation. It is likely that entropion is influenced by several genes (polygenic), defining the skin and other structures which make up the eyelids, the amount and weight of the skin covering the head and face, the orbital contents, and the conformation of the skull.

C.   Ectropion

A conformational defect resulting in eversion of the eyelids which may cause ocular irritation due to exposure. It is likely that ectropion is influenced by several genes (polygenic), defining the skin and other structures which make up the eyelids, the amount and weight of the skin covering the head and face, the orbital contents and the conformation of the skull.

D. Distichiasis

Eyelashes abnormally located in the eyelid margin which may cause ocular irritation. Distichiasis may occur at any time in the life of a dog. It is difficult to make a strong recommendation with regard to breeding dogs with this entity. The hereditary basis has not been established although it seems probable due to the high incidence in some breeds. Reducing the incidence is a logical goal. When diagnosed, distichiasis should be recorded; breeding discretion is advised.

E. Prolapse of the gland of the third eyelid

A protrusion of the tear gland associated with the third eyelid. The mode of inheritance of this disorder is unknown. The exposed gland may become irritated. Commonly referred to as "cherry eye".

F. Eversion of the cartilage of the third eyelid

A scroll-like curling of the cartilage of the third eyelid, usually everting the margin. This condition may occur in one or both eyes and may cause mild ocular irritation.

References

There are no references providing detailed descriptions of hereditary ocular conditions of the Saluki breed. The conditions listed above are generally recognized to exist in this breed, as evidenced by repeated references made in general texts.

1. ACVO Genetics Committee, 1992 and/or Data from CERF All-Breeds Report, 1991.

SAMOYED

	DISORDER	INHERITANCE	REFERENCE	BREEDING ADVICE
A.	Progressive Retinal Atrophy	Not defined	1	NO
B.	Cataract	Not defined	--	NO
C.	Corneal dystrophy	Not defined	--	Breeder option
D.	Glaucoma	Not defined	2	NO
E.	Distichiasis	Not defined	--	Breeder option
F.	Retinal dysplasia - focal/generalized w/ skeletal defects	Incomplete dominant	3,4	NO

Description and Comments

A.   Progressive Retinal Atrophy (PRA)

A degenerative disease of the retinal visual cells which may result in blindness. This abnormality may be detected by electroretinogram before it is apparent clinically. In all breeds studied to date, PRA is recessively inherited.

B.   Cataract

Lens opacity which may affect one or both eyes and may involve the lens partially or completely. In cases where cataracts are complete and affect both eyes, blindness results. The prudent approach is to assume cataracts to be hereditary except in cases known to be associated with trauma, other causes of ocular inflammation, specific metabolic diseases, persistent pupillary membranes, persistent hyaloid or nutritional deficiencies.

C.   Corneal dystrophy

A non-inflammatory corneal opacity (white to gray) present in one or more of the corneal layers; usually inherited and bilateral.

D.   Glaucoma

An elevation of intraocular pressure (IOP) which, when sustained, causes intraocular damage resulting in blindness. The elevated IOP occurs because the fluid cannot leave through the iridocorneal angle. Diagnosis and classification of glaucoma requires measurement of IOP (tonometry) and examination of the iridocorneal angle (gonioscopy). Neither of these tests are part of a routine breed eye screening exam.

E.   Distichiasis

Eyelashes abnormally located in the eyelid margin which may cause ocular irritation. Distichiasis may occur at any time in the life of a dog. It is difficult to make a strong recommendation with regard to breeding dogs with this entity. The hereditary basis has not been established, although it seems probable due to the high incidence in some breeds. Reducing the incidence is a logical goal. When diagnosed, distichiasis should be recorded; breeding discretion is advised.

F.   Retinal dysplasia - focal or generalized with skeletal defects

Abnormal development of the retina present at birth and recognized to have three forms:

        1) Retinal dysplasia - **folds**: linear, triangular, curved or curvilinear foci of retinal folding that may be single or multiple.
        2) Retinal dysplasia - **geographic**: any irregularly shaped area of abnormal retinal development, representing changes not accountable by simple folding.
        3) Retinal dysplasia - **detachment**: either of the above described forms of retinal dysplasia associated with separation (detachment) of the retina.

The two latter forms are associated with vision impairment or blindness. Retinal dysplasia is known to be inherited in many breeds. The genetic relationship between the three forms of the disease is not known for all breeds.

Based on studies of the Samoyed and a recent report of a limited family of dogs, retinal dysplasia in the Samoyed is an inherited defect similar to that reported in the Labrador retriever which affects the forelimb and the eye. The gene has recessive effects on the skeleton and incomplete dominant effects on the eye. Affected dogs are of small stature with valgus deformity of the carpi. Ocular abnormalities include cataract and retinal folds/multifocal retinal dysplasia and detachment. The gene responsible for the skeletal and ocular defects in the Samoyed is in the homozygous state and is in the heterozygous state for multiple retinal folds/multifocal retinal dysplasia. Some dogs may have focal/multifocal retinal dysplasia without skeletal defects.

Other Conditions Under Consideration

G. Uveitis associated with facial skin depigmentation (vitiligo) and hair depigmentation (poliosis)[5]

This form of uveitis is generally very severe. Adhesions between the iris and lens (posterior synechia) and the peripheral iris and cornea (peripheral anterior synechia) develop rapidly. Other complications include cataract development, retinal degeneration, retinal separation or detachment, optic disc atrophy and secondary glaucoma. Poliosis and/or vitiligo are generally later developments. This disorder is thought to represent an immune-mediated reaction to uveal and epidermal pigment cells. It appears to be similar to an oculocutaneous disorder in human patients known as the Vogt-Koyanagi-Harada syndrome. Some veterinary ophthalmologists feel there is a prevalence of this entity in the Samoyed. Additional studies are needed to validate this experience and explore the possibility of a genetic basis.

H. Vitreal degeneration

A liquefaction of the vitreous gel which may predispose to retinal detachment.

References

1. Dice PF: Progressive retinal atrophy in the Samoyed. Mod Vet Pract 1:59, 1980.

2. Wyman M, Ketring KL: Congenital glaucoma in the Basset hound: a biological model. Trans Am Acad Ophthalmol Otolaryngol 81: 645, 1976.

3. Meyers VN et al: Short-limbed dwarfism and ocular defects in the Samoyed dog. J Am Vet Med Assoc 183:975, 1983.

4. Acland GM, Aguirre GD: Retinal dysplasia in the Samoyed dog is the heterozygous phenotype of the gene (drd^s) for short-limbed dwarfism and ocular defects. Trans Amer College Vet Ophthalmol 22:44, 1991.

5. Bussanich MN et al: Granulomatous panuveitis and dermal depigmentation in dogs. J Am Anim Hosp Assoc 18:131, 1982.

SCHIPPERKE

	DISORDER	INHERITANCE	REFERENCE	BREEDING ADVICE
A.	Cataract	Not defined	--	NO
B.	Progressive Retinal Atrophy	Not defined	--	NO

Description and Comments

A.   Cataract

Lens opacity which may affect one or both eyes and may involve the lens partially or completely. In cases where cataracts are complete and affect both eyes, blindness results. The prudent approach is to assume cataracts to be hereditary except in cases known to be associated with trauma, other causes of ocular inflammation, specific metabolic diseases, persistent pupillary membranes, persistent hyaloid or nutritional deficiencies.

B.   Progressive Retinal Atrophy (PRA)

A degenerative disease of the retinal visual cells which progresses to blindness. This abnormality may be detected by electroretinogram before it is apparent clinically. In all breeds studied to date, PRA is recessively inherited.

References

There are no references providing detailed descriptions of hereditary ocular conditions of the Schipperke breed. The conditions listed above are generally recognized to exist in this breed, as evidenced by repeated references made in general texts.

1.   ACVO Genetics Committee, 1992 and/or Data from CERF All-Breeds Report, 1991.

SCOTTISH TERRIER

	DISORDER	INHERITANCE	REFERENCE	BREEDING ADVICE
A.	Cataract	Not defined	1	NO
B.	Luxated lens	Not defined	2	NO
C.	Progressive Retinal Atrophy	Not defined	1	NO
D.	Persistent pupillary membranes	Not defined	1	Breeder option

---

Description and Comments

A.   Cataract

Lens opacity which may affect one or both eyes and may involve the lens partially or completely. In cases where cataracts are complete and affect both eyes, blindness results. The prudent approach is to assume cataracts to be hereditary except in cases known to be associated with trauma, other causes of ocular inflammation, specific metabolic diseases, persistent pupillary membranes, persistent hyaloid or nutritional deficiencies.

B.   Luxated lens

Partial (subluxation) or complete displacement of the lens from the normal anatomic site behind the pupil. Lens luxation not associated with trauma or inflammation is presumed to be inherited. Lens luxation may result in elevated intraocular pressure (glaucoma), causing vision impairment or blindness.

C.   Progressive Retinal Atrophy (PRA)

A degenerative disease of the retinal visual cells which progresses to blindness. This abnormality may be detected by electroretinogram before it is apparent clinically. In all breeds studied to date, PRA is recessively inherited.

D.   Persistent pupillary membranes

Persistent blood vessel remnants in the anterior chamber of the eye which fail to regress normally in the neonatal period. These strands may bridge from iris to iris, iris to cornea, iris to lens, or form sheets of tissue in the anterior chamber. The last three forms pose the greatest threat to vision and when severe, vision impairment or blindness may occur.

References

There are no references providing detailed descriptions of hereditary ocular conditions of the Scottish Terrier breed. The conditions listed above are generally recognized to exist in this breed, as evidenced by repeated references made in general texts.

1.   ACVO Genetics Committee, 1992 and/or Data from CERF All-Breeds Report, 1991.

SEALYHAM TERRIER

	DISORDER	INHERITANCE	REFERENCE	BREEDING ADVICE
A.	Cataract	Not defined	1	NO
B.	Luxated lens	Not defined	1	NO
C.	Imperforate lacrimal punctum	Not defined	1	Breeder option
D.	Retinal dysplasia	Autosomal recessive	2,3	NO
E.	Progressive Retinal Atrophy	Not defined	1	NO

Description and Comments

A.   Cataract

Lens opacity which may affect one or both eyes and may involve the lens partially or completely. In cases where cataracts are complete and affect both eyes, blindness results. The prudent approach is to assume cataracts to be hereditary except in cases known to be associated with trauma, other causes of ocular inflammation, specific metabolic diseases, persistent pupillary membranes, persistent hyaloid or nutritional deficiencies.

B.   Luxated lens

Partial (subluxation) or complete displacement of the lens from the normal anatomic site behind the pupil. Lens luxation not associated with trauma or inflammation is presumed to be inherited. Lens luxation may result in elevated intraocular pressure (glaucoma) causing vision impairment or blindness.

C.   Imperforate lacrimal punctum

A developmental anomaly resulting in failure of opening of the lacrimal duct adjacent to the eye. The lower punctum is more frequently affected. This defect usually results in epiphora, an overflow of tears onto the face.

D.   Retinal dysplasia

Abnormal development of the retina present at birth and recognized to have three forms:

   1) Retinal dysplasia - **folds**: linear, triangular, curved or curvilinear foci of retinal folding that may be single or multiple.
   2) Retinal dysplasia - **geographic**: any irregularly shaped area of abnormal retinal development, representing changes not accountable by simple folding.
   3) Retinal dysplasia - **detachment**: either of the above described forms of retinal dysplasia associated with separation (detachment) of the retina.

The two latter forms are associated with vision impairment or blindness. Retinal dysplasia is known to be inherited in many breeds. The genetic relationship between the three forms of the disease is not known for all breeds.

E.   Progressive Retinal Atrophy (PRA)

A degenerative disease of the retinal visual cells which progresses to blindness. This abnormality may be detected by electroretinogram before it is apparent clinically. In all breeds studied to date, PRA is recessively inherited.

References

There are no references providing detailed descriptions of hereditary ocular conditions of the Sealyham Terrier breed. The conditions listed above are generally recognized to exist in this breed, as evidenced by repeated references made in general texts.

1.   ACVO Genetics Committee, 1992 and/or Data from CERF All-Breeds Report, 1991.

SHAR-PEI

	DISORDER	INHERITANCE	REFERENCE	BREEDING ADVICE
A.	Entropion	Not defined	1-3	NO
B.	Prolapsed gland of third eyelid	Not defined	4	Breeder option
C.	Lens luxation	Not defined	4	NO
D.	Progressive Retinal Atrophy	Not defined	4	NO
E.	Glaucoma	Not defined	4	NO

Description and Comments

A.   Entropion

A conformational defect resulting in an "in-rolling" of one or more of the eyelids which may cause ocular irritation. It is likely that entropion is influenced by several genes (polygenic), defining the skin and other structures which make up the eyelids, the amount and weight of the skin covering the head and face, the orbital contents, and the conformation of the skull.

The condition is a particularly severe problem in the Shar-Pei and is compounded by breeder selection for facial conformation which encourages formation of entropion.

B.   Prolapse of the gland of the third eyelid

Protrusion of the tear gland associated with the third eyelid. The mode of inheritance of this disorder is unknown. The exposed gland may become irritated. Commonly referred to as "cherry eye".

C.   Lens luxation

Partial (subluxation) or complete displacement of the lens from the normal anatomic site behind the pupil. Lens luxation not associated with trauma or inflammation is presumed to be inherited. Lens luxation may result in elevated intraocular pressure (glaucoma) causing vision impairment or blindness.

D.   Progressive Retinal Atrophy (PRA)

A degenerative disease of the retinal visual cells which progresses to blindness. This abnormality may be detected by electroretinogram before it is apparent clinically. In all breeds studied to date, PRA is recessively inherited.

E.   Glaucoma

Glaucoma is characterized by an elevation of intraocular pressure (IOP) which, when sustained, causes intraocular damage resulting in blindness. The elevated IOP occurs because the fluid cannot leave through the iridocorneal angle. Diagnosis and classification of glaucoma requires measurement of the intraocular pressure (tonometry) and examination of the iridocorneal angle (gonioscopy). Neither of these tests are part of a routine breed eye screening exam.

Other Conditions Under Consideration

F.   Cataract

Lens opacity which may affect one or both eyes and may involve the lens partially or completely. In cases where cataracts are complete and affect both eyes, blindness results. The prudent approach is to assume cataracts to be hereditary except in cases known to be associated with trauma, other causes of ocular inflammation, specific metabolic diseases, persistent pupillary membranes, persistent hyaloid or nutritional deficiencies.

References

1.   Lenarduzzi R: Management of eyelid problems in Chinese Shar-Pei puppies. Vet Med Small Anim Clin 78:548, 1983.

2.   Bedford PGC: Entropion in Shar Peis (Correspondence). Vet Rec 115:666, 1984.

3.   Startup FG: Entropion in the Shar Pei (Correspondence) Vet Rec 116:57, 1985.

4.   ACVO Genetics Committee, 1992 and/or Data from CERF All-Breeds Report, 1991.

SHETLAND SHEEPDOG

	DISORDER	INHERITANCE	REFERENCE	BREEDING ADVICE
A.	Distichiasis	Not defined	1	Breeder option
B.	Persistent pupillary membrane	Not defined	1	Breeder option
C.	Corneal dystrophy	Not defined	1,2	NO
D.	Choroidal hypoplasia	Not defined	1,2	NO
E.	Coloboma/ Staphyloma	Not defined	1,2	NO
F.	Progressive Retinal Atrophy	Not defined	1	NO
G.	Cataract	Not defined	1	NO

Description and Comments

A.   Distichiasis

Eyelashes abnormally located in the eyelid margin which may cause ocular irritation. Distichiasis may occur at any time in the life of a dog. It is difficult to make a strong recommendation with regard to breeding dogs with this entity. The hereditary basis has not been established although it seems probable due to the high incidence in some breeds. Reducing the incidence is a logical goal. When diagnosed, distichiasis should be recorded; breeding discretion is advised.

Distichiasis in the Shetland Sheepdog usually involves stiff hairs which require surgical removal.

B. Persistent pupillary membranes (PPM)

Persistent blood vessel remnants in the anterior chamber of the eye which fail to regress normally in the neonatal period. These strands may bridge from iris to iris, iris to cornea, iris to lens, or form sheets of tissue in the anterior chamber. The last three forms pose the greatest threat to vision and when severe, vision impairment or blindness may occur.

C. Corneal dystrophy

A non-inflammatory corneal opacity (white to gray) present in one or more of the corneal layers; usually inherited and bilateral.

The corneal changes in the Shetland Sheepdog are characterized grossly by multifocal, central, subepithelial and superficial stromal, grey-white, circular or irregular rings. Some affected animals develop corneal erosions. The preocular tear film in the majority of dogs is unstable and requires symptomatic therapy to keep the patients comfortable. Further studies are necessary to define this disorder.

D. Choroidal hypoplasia

An inadequate development of the choroid, present at birth. It does not progress as the dog ages.

E. Coloboma/Staphyloma

A coloboma is a congenital cleft or defect. A staphyloma is an area of scleral thinning lined by uveal tissue.

These two observed conditions are similar to those observed in the Collie Eye Anomaly, but to date retinal detachment and hemorrhage have not been observed in the Shetland Sheepdogs born, bred and raised in the U.S. Further studies are necessary to clarify the heritability of these anomalies in the Shetland Sheepdog.

F. Progressive Retinal Atrophy (PRA)

A degenerative disease of the retinal visual cells which progresses to blindness. This abnormality may be detected by electroretinogram before it is apparent clinically. In all breeds studied to date, PRA is recessively inherited.

G. Cataract

Lens opacity which may affect one or both eyes and may involve the lens partially or completely. In cases where cataracts are complete and affect both eyes, blindness results. The prudent approach is to assume cataracts to be hereditary except in cases known to be associated with trauma, other causes of ocular inflammation, specific metabolic diseases, persistent pupillary membrane, persistent hyaloid or nutritional deficiencies.

Other Conditions Under Consideration

H.   Optic nerve coloboma (without choroidal hypoplasia)

A congenital cavity in the optic nerve which, if large, may cause blindness or vision impairment.

References

1.   ACVO Genetics Committee, 1992 and/or Data from CERF All-Breeds Report, 1991.

2.   Dice P: Corneal dystrophy in the Shetland Sheepdog. Trans Am Coll Vet Ophthalmol 15:241, 1984.

SHIH TZU

	DISORDER	INHERITANCE	REFERENCE	BREEDING ADVICE
A.	Distichiasis	Not defined	1	Breeder option
B.	Ectopic cilia	Not defined	1	Breeder option
C.	Cataract	Not defined	1	NO
D.	Exposure keratopathy	Not defined	1	Breeder option
E.	Progressive Retinal Atrophy	Not defined	1	NO

Description and Comments

A.   Distichiasis

Eyelashes abnormally located in the eyelid margin which may cause ocular irritation. Distichiasis may occur at any time in the life of a dog. It is difficult to make a strong recommendation with regard to breeding dogs with this entity. The hereditary basis has not been established although it seems probable due to the high incidence in some breeds. Reducing the incidence is a logical goal. When diagnosed, distichiasis should be recorded; breeding discretion is advised.

B.   Ectopic cilia

Hair emerging through the eyelid conjunctiva. Ectopic cilia occur more frequently in younger dogs and cause discomfort and corneal disease.

C.   Cataract

Lens opacity which may affect one or both eyes and may involve the lens partially or completely. In cases where cataracts are complete and affect both eyes, blindness results. The prudent approach is to assume cataracts to be hereditary except in cases known to be associated with trauma, other causes of ocular inflammation, specific metabolic diseases, persistent pupillary membranes, persistent hyaloid or nutritional deficiencies.

D.   Exposure keratopathy syndrome

A corneal disease involving all or part of the cornea, resulting from inadequate blinking. This results from a combination of anatomic features including shallow orbits, exophthalmos, macroblepharon and lagophthalmos.

E.   Progressive Retinal Atrophy (PRA)

A degenerative disease of the retinal visual cells which progresses to blindness. This abnormality may be detected by electroretinogram before it is apparent clinically. In all breeds studied to date, PRA is recessively inherited.

Other Conditions Under Consideration

F.   Dry eye

An abnormality of the tear film, most commonly a deficiency of the aqueous portion, although the mucin and/or lipid layers may be affected; results in ocular irritation and/or vision impairment.

G.   Retinal detachment

The separation of the sensory retina from the underlying tissue. It results in blindness when complete.

H.   Ciliated caruncle

Fleshy conjunctival tissue at the nasal canthus; may contain hair (ciliated caruncle) which, if contacting the cornea, may cause irritation and/or tearing.

I.   Lagophthalmos

Failure to close the eyelids completely; results in exposure of the cornea and conjunctiva.

J.   Optic nerve hypoplasia

A congenital defect of the optic nerve which causes blindness and abnormal pupil response in the affected eye. May be unable to differentiate from micropapilla on a routine (dilated) screening ophthalmoscopic exam.

References

1.   ACVO Genetics Committee, 1992 and/or Data from CERF All-Breeds Report, 1991.

SIBERIAN HUSKY

	DISORDER	INHERITANCE	REFERENCE	BREEDING ADVICE
A.	Progressive Retinal Atrophy	Not defined	--	NO
B.	Cataract	Not defined	1	NO
C.	Corneal dystrophy	Autosomal recessive	2	NO
D.	Glaucoma	Not defined	3	NO
E.	Entropion	Not defined	--	Breeder option

Description and Comments

A. Progressive Retinal Atrophy (PRA)

A degenerative disease of the retinal visual cells which progresses to blindness. This abnormality may be detected by electroretinogram before it is apparent clinically. In all breeds studied to date, PRA is recessively inherited.

B. Cataract

Lens opacity which may affect one or both eyes and may involve the lens partially or completely. In cases where cataracts are complete and affect both eyes, blindness results. The prudent approach is to assume cataracts to be hereditary except in cases known to be associated with trauma, other causes of ocular inflammation, specific metabolic diseases, persistent pupillary membranes, persistent hyaloid or nutritional deficiencies.

C. Corneal dystrophy

A non-inflammatory corneal opacity (white to gray) present in one or more of the corneal layers; usually inherited and bilateral.

257

D.   Glaucoma

An elevation of intraocular pressure (IOP) which, when sustained, causes intraocular damage resulting in blindness. The elevated IOP occurs because the fluid cannot leave through the iridocorneal angle. Diagnosis and classification of glaucoma requires measurement of IOP (tonometry) and examination of the iridocorneal angle (gonioscopy). Neither of these tests are part of a routine breed eye screening exam.

E.   Entropion

A conformational defect resulting in an "in-rolling" of one or more of the eyelids which may cause ocular irritation. It is likely that entropion is influenced by several genes (polygenic), defining the skin and other structures which make up the eyelids, the amount and weight of the skin covering the head and face, the orbital contents, and the conformation of the skull.

Other Conditions Under Consideration

F.   Uveitis associated with facial skin depigmentation (vitiligo) and hair depigmentation (poliosis)

This form of uveitis is generally very severe. Adhesions between the iris and lens (posterior synechia) and the peripheral iris and cornea (peripheral anterior synechia) develop rapidly. Other complications include cataract development, retinal degeneration, retinal separation or detachment, optic disc atrophy and secondary glaucoma. Poliosis and/or vitiligo are generally later developments. This disorder is thought to represent an immune-mediated reaction to uveal and epidermal pigment cells. It appears to be similar to an oculocutaneous disorder in human patients known as the Vogt-Koyanagi-Harada syndrome.

Some veterinary ophthalmologists feel there is a prevalence of this entity in the Siberian Husky. Additional studies are needed to validate this experience and explore the possibility of a genetic basis.

G.   Uveitis (without vitiligo or poliosis)

Some veterinary ophthalmologists feel that uveitis without skin or hair depigmentation may occur with greater frequency in the Siberian Husky than in most other breeds. At this time, adequate documentation is lacking.

References

1. MacMillan A: Unpublished.

2. Waring GO et al: Inheritance of crystalline corneal dystrophy in Siberian Huskies. J Am Anim Hosp Assoc 22:655, 1986.

3. Wyman M, Ketring KL: Congenital glaucoma in the Basset hound: A biologic model. Trans Am Acad Ophthalmol Otolaryngol 81:645, 1976.

4. Halliwell REW: Autoimmune diseases in domestic animals. J Am Vet Med Assoc 181:1088, 1982.

5. Bussanich MN et al: Granulomatous panuveitis and dermal depigmentation in dogs. J Am Anim Hosp Assoc 18:131, 1982.

SILKY TERRIER

	DISORDER	INHERITANCE	REFERENCE	BREEDING ADVICE
A.	Cataract	Not defined	1	NO
B.	Progressive Retinal Atrophy	Not defined	1	NO

Description and Comments

A.   Cataract

Lens opacity which may affect one or both eyes and may involve the lens partially or completely. In cases where cataracts are complete and affect both eyes, blindness results. The prudent approach is to assume cataracts to be hereditary except in cases known to be associated with trauma, other causes of ocular inflammation, specific metabolic diseases, persistent pupillary membranes, persistent hyaloid or nutritional deficiencies.

B.   Progressive Retinal Atrophy (PRA)

A degenerative disease of the retinal visual cells which progresses to blindness. This abnormality may be detected by electroretinogram before it is apparent clinically. In all breeds studied to date, PRA is recessively inherited.

References

There are no references providing detailed descriptions of hereditary ocular conditions of the Silky Terrier breed. The conditions listed above are generally recognized to exist in this breed, as evidenced by repeated references made in general texts.

1.   ACVO Genetics Committee, 1992 and/or Data from CERF All-Breeds Report, 1991.

SOFT-COATED WHEATEN TERRIER

	DISORDER	INHERITANCE	REFERENCE	BREEDING ADVICE
A.	Persistent pupillary membranes	Not defined	--	Breeder option
B.	Cataract	Not defined	--	NO
C.	Progressive Retinal Atrophy	Not defined	--	NO

Description and Comments

A.   Persistent pupillary membranes (PPM)

Persistent blood vessel remnants in the anterior chamber of the eye which fail to regress normally in the neonatal period. These strands may bridge from iris to iris, iris to cornea, or form sheets of tissue in the anterior chamber. The last three forms pose the greatest threat to vision and when severe, vision impairment or blindness may occur.

B.   Cataract

Lens opacity which may affect one or both eyes and may involve the lens partially or completely. In cases where cataracts are complete and affect both eyes, blindness results. The prudent approach is to assume cataracts to be hereditary except in cases known to be associated with trauma, other causes of ocular inflammation, specific metabolic diseases, persistent pupillary membranes, persistent hyaloid or nutritional deficiencies.

C.   Progressive Retinal Atrophy (PRA)

A degenerative disease of the retinal visual cells which progresses to blindness. This abnormality may be detected by electroretinogram before it is apparent clinically. In all breeds studied to date, PRA is recessively inherited.

References

There are no references providing detailed descriptions of hereditary ocular conditions of the Soft-Coated Wheaten Terrier breed. The conditions listed are generally recognized to exist in this breed, as evidenced by repeated references made in general texts.

1.   ACVO Genetics Committee, 1992 and/or Data from CERF All-Breeds Report, 1991.

SPINONI ITALIANI

	DISORDER	INHERITANCE	REFERENCE	BREEDING ADVICE
A.	Ectropion	Not defined	1	Breeder option

Description and Comments

A.   Ectropion

A conformational defect resulting in eversion of the eyelids, which may cause ocular irritation due to exposure. It is likely that ectropion is influenced by several genes (polygenic) defining the skin and other structures which make up the eyelids, the amount and weight of the skin covering the head and face, the orbital contents and the conformation of the skull.

References

There are no references providing detailed descriptions of hereditary ocular conditions of the Spinoni Italiani breed. The condition listed is generally recognized to exist in the breed, as evidenced by repeated references made in general texts.

1.   ACVO Genetics Committee, 1992 and/or Data from CERF All-Breeds Report, 1991.

STAFFORDSHIRE BULL TERRIER (English)

	DISORDER	INHERITANCE	REFERENCE	BREEDING ADVICE
A.	Entropion	Not defined	1	Breeder option
B.	Hyperplastic primary vitreous	Not defined	2,3	NO
C.	Cataract	Not defined	4,5	NO

Description and Comments

A.   Entropion

A conformational defect resulting in an "in-rolling" of one or more of the eyelids which may cause ocular irritation. It is likely that entropion is influenced by several genes (polygenic), defining the skin and other structures which make up the eyelids, the amount and weight of the skin covering the head and face, the orbital contents, and the conformation of the skull.

C.   Cataract

Lens opacity which may affect one or both eyes and may involve the lens partially or completely. In cases where cataracts are complete and affect both eyes, blindness results. The prudent approach is to assume cataracts to be hereditary except in cases known to be associated with trauma, other causes of ocular inflammation, specific metabolic diseases, persistent pupillary membranes, persistent hyaloid or nutritional deficiencies.

Cataracts in the Staffordshire bull terrier have been reported to be similar to those in the Boston terrier, beginning in the first year, with progression to complete blindness within the first several years of life.

C.   Persistent hyperplastic primary vitreous (PHPV)

A congenital defect resulting from abnormalities in the development and regression of the hyaloid artery (the primary vitreous) and the interaction of this blood vessel with the posterior lens capsule/cortex during embryogenesis. This condition is often associated with **persistent tunica vasculosa lentis (PTVL)** which results from failure of regression of the embryologic vascular network which surrounds the developing lens.

References

1.   ACVO Genetics Committee, 1992 and/or Data from CERF All-Breeds Report, 1991.

2.   Curtis R, Barnett KC, Leon A: Persistent hyperplastic primary vitreous in the Staffordshire bull terrier. Vet Rec 115: 385, 1984.

3.   Leon A, Curtis B, Barnett KC: Hereditary persistent hyperplastic primary vitreous in the Staffordshire bull terrier. J Am Anim Hosp Assoc 22:765, 1986.

4.   Barnett KC: The diagnosis and differential diagnosis of cataracts in the dog. J Small Anim Pract 26:305, 1985.

5.   Barnett KC: Hereditary cataract in the dog. J Small Anim Pract 19:109, 1978.

STANDARD SCHNAUZER

	DISORDER	INHERITANCE	REFERENCE	BREEDING ADVICE
A.	Cataract	Not defined	--	NO
B.	Retinal dysplasia - folds	Not defined	--	Breeder option

Description and Comments

A. Cataract

Lens opacity which may affect one or both eyes and may involve the lens partially or completely. In cases where cataracts are complete and affect both eyes, blindness results. The prudent approach is to assume cataracts to be hereditary except in cases known to be associated with trauma, other causes of ocular inflammation, specific metabolic diseases, persistent pupillary membranes, persistent hyaloid or nutritional deficiencies.

There are apparently several forms of cataract in the breed: 1) posterior cortex and posterior/total nucleus involvement, with slow progression; 2) dense posterior polar opacity near the subcapsular region which progresses rapidly to very dense posterior polar plaques in young animals; 3) dense posterior polar opacity like that reported in young animals but found in older animals with variable progression.

B. Retinal dysplasia

Abnormal development of the retina present at birth and recognized to have three forms:

1) Retinal dysplasia - **folds**: linear, triangular, curved or curvilinear foci of retinal folding that may be single or multiple.
2) Retinal dysplasia - **geographic**: any irregularly shaped area of abnormal retinal development, representing changes not accountable by simple folding.
3) Retinal dysplasia - **detachment**: either of the above described forms of retinal dysplasia associated with separation (detachment) of the retina.

266

The two latter forms are associated with vision impairment or blindness. Retinal dysplasia is known to be inherited in many breeds. The genetic relationship between the three forms of the disease is not known for all breeds.

Other Conditions Under Consideration

C.   Dry eye

An abnormality of the tear film, most commonly a deficiency of the aqueous portion, although the mucin and/or lipid layers may be affected; results in ocular irritation and/or vision impairment.

References

There are no references providing detailed descriptions of hereditary ocular conditions of the Standard Schnauzer breed. The conditions listed are generally recognized to exist in the breed, as evidenced by repeated references made in general texts.

1.   ACVO Genetics Committee, 1992 and/or Data from CERF All-Breeds Report, 1991.

SUSSEX SPANIEL

	DISORDER	INHERITANCE	REFERENCE	BREEDING ADVICE
A.	Entropion	Not defined	1,2	Breeder option
B.	Cataract	Not defined	1,2	NO
C.	Retinal dysplasia - folds	Not defined	1	Breeder option

Description and Comments

A.   Entropion

A conformational defect resulting in "in-rolling" of one or more of the eyelids which may cause ocular irritation. It is likely that entropion is influenced by several genes (polygenic), defining the skin and other structures which make up the eyelids, the amount and weight of the skin covering the head and face, the orbital contents and the conformation of the skull.

B.   Cataract

Lens opacity which may affect one or both eyes and may involve the lens partially or completely. In cases where cataracts are complete and affect both eyes, blindness results. The prudent approach is to assume cataracts to be hereditary except in cases known to be associated with trauma, other causes of ocular inflammation, specific metabolic diseases, persistent pupillary membrane, persistent hyaloid or nutritional deficiencies.

C.   Retinal dysplasia

Abnormal development of the retina present at birth and recognized to have three forms:

1) Retinal dysplasia - **folds**: linear, triangular, curved or curvilinear foci of retinal folding that may be single or multiple.
2) Retinal dysplasia - **geographic**: any irregularly shaped area of abnormal retinal development, representing changes not accountable by simple folding.

3) Retinal dysplasia - **detachment**: either of the above described forms of retinal dysplasia associated with separation (detachment) of the retina.

The two latter forms are associated with vision impairment or blindness. Retinal dysplasia is known to be inherited in many breeds. The genetic relationship between the three forms of the disease is not known for all breeds. Only multifocal folds have been reported in the Sussex Spaniel.

References

There are no references providing detailed descriptions of hereditary ocular conditions of the Sussex Spaniel breed. The conditions listed above are generally recognized to exist in this breed, as evidenced by repeated references made in general texts.

1.   ACVO Genetics Committee, 1992 and/or Data from CERF All-Breeds Report, 1991.

2.   Rubin LF: Inherited Eye Diseases in Purebred Dogs. Williams and Wilkins, Baltimore, 1989.

TIBETAN TERRIER

	DISORDER	INHERITANCE	REFERENCE	BREEDING ADVICE
A.	Progressive Retinal Atrophy	Not defined	1-4	NO
B.	Lens luxation	Autosomal recessive	5-7	NO
C.	Cataract	Not defined	--	NO
D.	Retinal dysplasia - geographic	Not defined	--	Breeder option

Description and Comments

A.   Progressive Retinal Atrophy (PRA)

A degenerative disease of the retinal visual cells which progresses to blindness. This abnormality may be detected by electroretinogram before it is apparent clinically. In all breeds studied to date, PRA is recessively inherited.

There are some reports to suggest there may be more than one variety of this disorder in the Tibetan Terrier:
1) Emerging night blindness at 1-2 years of age (up to 1-4 years of age), with ophthalmoscopic signs of peripheral to central retinal atrophy emerging soon thereafter.
2) Individuals with advanced night blindness at a younger age but with no obvious ophthalmoscopic signs until perhaps 4 years of age.

There are ERG studies to indicate that there is depression of the B wave at 10-12 weeks of age in the second variety and slower depression in the first variety. Some may have no obvious signs at 5-6 years of age, only to develop clinical signs at 6-7 years of age. It is logical that any animal found with signs of bilateral atrophy should not be bred. Members of the family of the affected animal should be carefully screened. Perhaps ERG in animals less than 4 years of age is logical, especially if the animal is intended for breed foundation.

B. Luxated lens

Partial (subluxation) or complete displacement of the lens from the normal anatomic site behind the pupil. Lens luxation not associated with trauma or inflammation is presumed to be inherited. Lens luxation may result in elevated intraocular pressure (glaucoma), causing vision impairment or blindness.

C. Cataract

Lens opacity which may affect one or both eyes and may involve the lens partially or completely. In cases where cataracts are complete and affect both eyes, blindness results. The prudent approach is to assume cataracts to be hereditary except in cases known to be associated with trauma, other causes of ocular inflammation, specific metabolic diseases, persistent pupillary membranes, persistent hyaloid or nutritional deficiencies.

D. Retinal dysplasia

Abnormal development of the retina present at birth and recognized to have three forms:

1) Retinal dysplasia - **folds**: linear, triangular, curved or curvilinear foci of retinal folding that may be single or multiple.
2) Retinal dysplasia - **geographic**: any irregularly shaped area of abnormal retinal development, representing changes not accountable by simple folding.
3) Retinal dysplasia - **detachment**: either of the above described forms of retinal dysplasia associated with separation (detachment) of the retina.

The two latter forms are associated with vision impairment or blindness. Retinal dysplasia is known to be inherited in many breeds. The genetic relationship between the three forms of the disease is not known for all breeds.

Other Conditions Under Consideration

E. Persistent hyperplastic primary vitreous (PHPV)

A congenital defect resulting from abnormalities in the development and regression of the hyaloid artery (the primary vitreous) and the interaction of this blood vessel with the posterior lens capsule/cortex during embryogenesis. This condition is often associated with persistent tunica vasculosa lentis (PTVL) which results from failure of regression of the embryologic network which surrounds the developing lens.

References

1.   Riis R, Loew E: Tibetan terrier retinopathy update. Trans Am Coll Vet Ophthalmol, 1985.

2.   Loew E, Riis R: Congenital nyctalopia in the Tibetan terrier. Trans Am Coll Vet Ophthalmol, 1983.

3.   Millichamp N et al: Progressive retinal atrophy in the Tibetan terrier. J Am Vet Med Assoc 192:769, 1987.

4.   ACVO Genetics Committee, 1992 and/or Data from CERF All-Breeds Report, 1991.

5.   Willis MB et al: Genetic aspects of lens luxation in the Tibetan terrier. Vet Rec 104:409, 1979.

6.   Barnett KC, Curtis R: Lens luxation and progressive retinal atrophy in the Tibetan terrier. Vet Rec 103:160, 1978.

7.   Curtis R, Barnett KC: Primary lens luxation in the dog. J Small Anim Pract 21:257, 1980.

VIZSLA

	DISORDER	INHERITANCE	REFERENCE	BREEDING ADVICE
A.	Entropion	Not defined	1	Breeder option
B.	Cataract	Not defined	1	NO
C.	Progressive Retinal Atrophy	Not defined	1	NO

Description and Comments

A. Entropion

A conformational defect resulting in an "in-rolling" of one or more of the eyelids which may cause ocular irritation. It is likely that entropion is influenced by several genes (polygenic), defining the skin and other structures which make up the eyelids, the amount and weight of the skin covering the head and face, the orbital contents, and the conformation of the skull.

B. Cataract

Lens opacity which may affect one or both eyes and may involve the lens partially or completely. In cases where cataracts are complete and affect both eyes, blindness results. The prudent approach is to assume cataracts to be hereditary except in cases known to be associated with trauma, other causes of ocular inflammation, specific metabolic diseases, persistent pupillary membranes, persistent hyaloid or nutritional deficiencies.

C. Progressive Retinal Atrophy (PRA)

A degenerative disease of the retinal visual cells which progresses to blindness. This abnormality may be detected by electroretinogram before it is apparent clinically. In all breeds studied to date, PRA is recessively inherited.

273

Other Conditions Under Consideration

D.   Corneal Dystrophy

A non-inflammatory corneal opacity (white to gray) present in one or more of the corneal layers; usually inherited and bilateral.

References

There are no references providing detailed descriptions of hereditary ocular conditions of the Vizsla breed. The conditions listed above are generally recognized to exist in this breed, as evidenced by repeated references made in general texts.

1.   ACVO Genetics Committee, 1992 and/or Data from CERF All-Breeds Report, 1991.

WEIMARANER

	DISORDER	INHERITANCE	REFERENCE	BREEDING ADVICE
A.	Distichiasis	Not defined	1	Breeder option
B.	Entropion	Not defined	1	Breeder option
C.	Everted cartilage of third eyelid	Not defined	1	Breeder option

Description and Comments

A. Distichiasis

Eyelashes abnormally located in the eyelid margin which may cause ocular irritation. Distichiasis may occur at any time in the life of a dog. It is difficult to make a strong recommendation with regard to breeding dogs with this entity. The hereditary basis has not been established although it seems probable due to the high incidence in some breeds. Reducing the incidence is a logical goal. When diagnosed, distichiasis should be recorded; breeding discretion is advised.

In this breed, because there is significant clinical disease associated with the abnormal hairs, breeding should be discouraged.

B. Entropion

A conformational defect resulting in an "in-rolling" of one or more of the eyelids which may cause ocular irritation. It is likely that entropion is influenced by several genes (polygenic), defining the skin and other structures which make up the eyelids, the amount and weight of the skin covering the head and face, the orbital contents, and the conformation of the skull.

C. Eversion of the cartilage of the third eyelid

A scroll-like curling of the cartilage of the third eyelid, usually everting the margin. This condition may occur in one or both eyes and may cause mild ocular irritation.

References

There are no references providing detailed descriptions of hereditary ocular conditions of the Weimaraner breed. The conditions listed are generally recognized to exist in the breed, as evidenced by repeated references made in general texts.

1.   ACVO Genetics Committee, 1992 and/or Data from CERF All-Breeds Report, 1991.

WELSH CORGI, CARDIGAN

	DISORDER	INHERITANCE	REFERENCE	BREEDING ADVICE
A.	Persistent pupillary membrane	Not defined	1	Breeder option
B.	Progressive Retinal Atrophy	Not defined	2	NO
C.	Central Progressive Retinal Atrophy	Not defined	3	NO
D.	Retinal dysplasia - focal/multifocal	Not defined	1	Breeder option

Description and Comments

A.   Persistent pupillary membranes

Persistent blood vessel remnants in the anterior chamber of the eye which fail to regress normally in the neonatal period. These strands may bridge from iris to iris, iris to cornea, iris to lens, or form sheets of tissue in the anterior chamber. The last three forms pose the greatest threat to vision and when severe, vision impairment or blindness may occur.

B.   Progressive Retinal Atrophy (PRA)

A degenerative disease of the retinal visual cells which progresses to blindness. This abnormality may be detected by electroretinogram before it is apparent clinically. In all breeds studied to date, PRA is recessively inherited.

In the Cardigan Welsh Corgi, PRA begins early in life, and clinical signs may be seen as early as 6-8 weeks of age.

C. Central Progressive Retinal Atrophy (CPRA)

A progressive retinal degeneration in which photoreceptor death occurs secondary to disease of the underlying pigment epithelium. Progression is slow and some animals never lose vision. CPRA occurs in England, but is uncommon elsewhere.

D. Retinal dysplasia

Abnormal development of the retina present at birth and recognized to have three forms:

1) Retinal dysplasia - **folds**: linear, triangular, curved or curvilinear foci of retinal folding that may be single or multiple.
2) Retinal dysplasia - **geographic**: any irregularly shaped area of abnormal retinal development, representing changes not accountable by simple folding.
3) Retinal dysplasia - **detachment**: either of the above described forms of retinal dysplasia associated with separation (detachment) of the retina.

The two latter forms are associated with vision impairment or blindness. Retinal dysplasia is known to be inherited in many breeds. The genetic relationship between the three forms of the disease is not known for all breeds.

References

1. ACVO Genetics Committee, 1992 and/or Data from CERF All-Breeds Report, 1991.

2. Barnett KC: Comparative aspects of canine hereditary eye disease. Adv Vet Sc Comp Med 20:39, 1976.

3. Keep JM: Clinical aspects of progressive retinal atrophy in the Cardigan Welsh Corgi. Aust Vet J 48:197, 1972.

WELSH CORGI, PEMBROKE

	DISORDER	INHERITANCE	REFERENCE	BREEDING ADVICE
A.	Persistent pupillary membranes	Not defined	1	Breeder option
B.	Cataract	Not defined	1	NO
C.	Progressive Retinal Atrophy	Not defined	1	NO
D.	Retinal dysplasia - geographic	Not defined	1	Breeder option

Description and Comments

A.   Persistent pupillary membranes (PPM)

Persistent blood vessel remnants in the anterior chamber of the eye which fail to regress normally in the neonatal period. These strands may bridge from iris to iris, iris to cornea, iris to lens, or form sheets of tissue in the anterior chamber. The last three forms pose the greatest threat to vision and when severe, vision impairment or blindness may occur.

B.   Cataract

Lens opacity which may affect one or both eyes and may involve the lens partially or completely. In cases where cataracts are complete and affect both eyes, blindness results. The prudent approach is to assume cataracts to be hereditary except in cases known to be associated with trauma, other causes of ocular inflammation, specific metabolic diseases, persistent pupillary membranes, persistent hyaloid or nutritional deficiencies.

C.   Progressive Retinal Atrophy (PRA)

A degenerative disease of the retinal visual cells which progresses to blindness. This abnormality may be detected by electroretinogram before it is apparent clinically. In all breeds studied to date, PRA is recessively inherited.

D.   Retinal dysplasia

Abnormal development of the retina present at birth and recognized to have three forms:

1) Retinal dysplasia - **folds**: linear, triangular, curved or curvilinear foci of retinal folding that may be single or multiple.
2) Retinal dysplasia - **geographic**: any irregularly shaped area of abnormal retinal development, representing changes not accountable by simple folding.
3) Retinal dysplasia - **detachment**: either of the above described forms of retinal dysplasia associated with separation (detachment) of the retina.

The two latter forms are associated with vision impairment or blindness. Retinal dysplasia is known to be inherited in many breeds. The genetic relationship between the three forms of the disease is not known for all breeds.

References

There are no specific references providing detailed descriptions of hereditary ocular conditions of the Pembroke Welsh Corgi breed. The conditions listed above are generally recognized to exist in this breed, as evidenced by repeated references made in general texts.

1.   ACVO Genetics Committee, 1992 and/or Data from CERF All-Breeds Report, 1991.

WELSH SPRINGER SPANIEL

	DISORDER	INHERITANCE	REFERENCE	BREEDING ADVICE
A.	Cataract	Autosomal recessive	1	NO
B.	Progressive Retinal Atrophy	Not defined	2	NO
C.	Glaucoma	Autosomal dominant	3	NO

Description and Comments

A.   Cataract

Lens opacity which may affect one or both eyes and may involve the lens partially or completely. In cases where cataracts are complete and affect both eyes, blindness results. The prudent approach is to assume cataracts to be hereditary except in cases known to be associated with trauma, other causes of ocular inflammation, specific metabolic diseases, persistent pupillary membrane, persistent hyaloid or nutritional deficiencies. Lesions may be seen as early as 8-12 weeks of age and progress rapidly to complete cataract, impairing vision. A recessive mode of inheritance is reported.

B.   Progressive Retinal Atrophy (PRA)

A degenerative disease of the retinal visual cells which progresses to blindness. This abnormality may be detected by electroretinogram before it is apparent clinically. In all breeds studied to date, PRA is recessively inherited. Clinical onset is 5 to 7 years of age.

C.   Glaucoma

An elevation of intraocular pressure (IOP) which, when sustained, causes intraocular damage resulting in blindness. The elevated IOP occurs because the fluid cannot leave through the iridocorneal angle. Diagnosis and classification of glaucoma requires measurement of IOP (tonometry) and examination of the iridocorneal angle (gonioscopy). Neither of these tests are part of a routine breed eye screening exam.

Primary angle closure glaucoma has been reported in the Welsh Springer Spaniel. Females are affected more than males. Onset ranges from 10 weeks to 10 years. At the iridocorneal angle, the pectinate ligaments appear sparse and wispy in contrast to the sturdy fibers seen in other breeds. A dominant mode of inheritance is reported.

References

1.   Barnett KC: Hereditary cataract in the Welsh springer spaniel. J Small Anim Pract 21: 621, 1980.

2.   Priester WA: Canine progressive retinal atrophy. Occurrence by age, breed and sex. Am J Vet Res 35: 571, 1974.

3.   Cottrell BD: Primary glaucoma in the Welsh springer spaniel. Trans Am Coll Vet Ophthalmol 1986, pp 155-176.

WELSH TERRIER

	DISORDER	INHERITANCE	REFERENCE	BREEDING ADVICE
A.	Glaucoma	Not defined	1	NO
B.	Luxated Lens	Not defined	1	NO

Description and Comments

A.   Glaucoma

Glaucoma is characterized by an elevation of intraocular pressure (IOP) which, when sustained, causes intraocular damage resulting in blindness. The elevated IOP occurs because the fluid cannot leave through the iridocorneal angle. Diagnosis and classification of glaucoma requires measurement of IOP (tonometry) and examination of the iridocorneal angle (gonioscopy). Neither of these tests are part of a routine breed eye screening exam.

B.   Luxated lens

Partial (subluxation) or complete displacement of the lens from the normal anatomic site behind the pupil. Lens luxation not associated with trauma or inflammation is presumed to be inherited. Lens luxation may result in elevated intraocular pressure (glaucoma) causing vision impairment or blindness.

References

There are no references providing detailed descriptions of hereditary ocular conditions of the Welsh Terrier. The conditions listed are generally recognized to exist in the breed, as evidenced by repeated references made in general texts.

1.   ACVO Genetics Committee, 1992 and/or Data from CERF All-Breeds Report, 1991.

WEST HIGHLAND WHITE TERRIER

	DISORDER	INHERITANCE	REFERENCE	BREEDING ADVICE
A.	Dry eye	Not defined	1-4	NO
B.	Cataract	Autosomal recessive	5	NO

Description and Comments

A.   Dry eye

An abnormality of the tear film, most commonly a deficiency of the aqueous portion, although the mucin and/or lipid layers may be affected; results in ocular irritation and/or vision impairment.

B.   Cataract

Lens opacity which may affect one or both eyes and may involve the lens partially or completely. In cases where cataracts are complete and affect both eyes, blindness results. The prudent approach is to assume cataracts to be hereditary except in cases known to be associated with trauma, other causes of ocular inflammation, specific metabolic diseases, persistent pupillary membranes, persistent hyaloid or nutritional deficiencies.

The cataract described in this breed involves the posterior Y sutures and may infrequently progress, resulting in vision impairment. A recessive mode of inheritance is suggested by the pedigrees which have been studied.

References

1.   Sansom J, Barnett KC: Keratoconjunctivitis sicca in the dog: A review of two hundred cases. J Sm Anim Pract 26:121, 1985.

2.   Baker GJ, Formston C: Evaluation of transplantation of the parotid duct in the treatment of keratoconjunctivitis sicca. J Sm Anim Pract 9:261, 1968.

3. Kaswan RL, Martin CL, Chapman WL: Keratoconjunctivitis sicca: Histopathologic study of the nictitating membrane and lacrimal glands from 28 dogs. Am J Vet Res 45:112, 1984.

4. Helper LC: Trans Am Acad Ophthalmol and Otolaryngol, 1976.

5. Narfstrom K: Cataract in the West Highland White terrier. J Sm Anim Pract 22:467, 1981.

WHIPPET

	DISORDER	INHERITANCE	REFERENCE	BREEDING ADVICE
A.	Cataract	Not defined	1,2	NO
B.	Progressive Retinal Atrophy	Not defined	1	NO
C.	Vitreal degeneration	Not defined	1	Breeder option
D.	Lens luxation	Not defined	1	NO

Description and Comments

A.   Cataract

Lens opacity which may affect one or both eyes and may involve the lens partially or completely. In cases where cataracts are complete and affect both eyes, blindness results. The prudent approach is to assume cataracts to be hereditary except in cases known to be associated with trauma, other causes of ocular inflammation, specific metabolic diseases, persistent pupillary membranes, persistent hyaloid or nutritional deficiencies.

B.   Progressive Retinal Atrophy (PRA)

A degenerative disease of the retinal visual cells which progresses to blindness. This abnormality may be detected by electroretinogram before it is apparent clinically. In all breeds studied to date, PRA is recessively inherited.

C.   Vitreal degeneration

A liquefaction of the vitreous gel which may predispose to retinal detachment.

D.   Lens luxation

Partial (subluxation) or complete displacement of the lens from the normal anatomic site behind the pupil. Lens luxation not associated with trauma or inflammation is presumed to be inherited. Lens luxation may result in elevated intraocular pressure (glaucoma) causing vision impairment or blindness.

References

There are no references providing detailed descriptions of hereditary ocular conditions of the Whippet breed. The conditions listed above are generally recognized to exist in this breed, as evidenced by repeated references made in general texts.

1. ACVO Genetics Committee, 1992 and/or Data from CERF All-Breeds Report, 1991.

2. Rubin LF: <u>Inherited Eye Diseases in Purebred Dogs</u>. Baltimore: Williams & Wilkins, 1989.

YORKSHIRE TERRIER

	DISORDER	INHERITANCE	REFERENCE	BREEDING ADVICE
A.	Entropion	Not defined	1	Breeder option
B.	Dry eye	Not defined	1	NO
C.	Cataract	Not defined	1	NO
D.	Progressive Retinal Atrophy	Not defined	1	NO

Description and Comments

A.   Entropion

A conformational defect resulting in an "in-rolling" of one or more of the eyelids which may cause ocular irritation. It is likely that entropion is influenced by several genes (polygenic), defining the skin and other structures which make up the eyelids, the amount and weight of the skin covering the head and face, the orbital contents, and the conformation of the skull. In this breed, the inner portions of the eyelid are most frequently affected and tearing is the most prominent sign.

B.   Dry eye

An abnormality of the tear film, most commonly a deficiency of the aqueous portion, although the mucin and/or lipid layers may be affected; results in ocular irritation and/or vision impairment.

C.   Cataract

Lens opacity which may affect one or both eyes and may involve the lens partially or completely. In cases where cataracts are complete and affect both eyes, blindness results. The prudent approach is to assume cataracts to be hereditary except in cases known to be associated with trauma, other causes of ocular inflammation, specific metabolic diseases, persistent pupillary membranes, persistent hyaloid or nutritional deficiencies.

D.   Progressive Retinal Atrophy (PRA)

A degenerative disease of the retinal visual cells which progresses to blindness. This abnormality may be detected by electroretinogram before it is apparent clinically. In all breeds studied to date, PRA is recessively inherited.

References

There are no references providing detailed descriptions of hereditary ocular conditions of the Yorkshire Terrier. The conditions listed above are generally recognized to exist in the breed, as evidenced by repeated references made in general texts.

1.   ACVO Genetics Committee, 1992 and/or Data from CERF All-Breeds Report, 1991.

OCULAR DISORDERS
PROVEN OR SUSPECTED TO BE HEREDITARY IN DOGS

by the GENETICS COMMITTEE of the

AMERICAN COLLEGE of VETERINARY OPHTHALMOLOGISTS

To order extra copies of this book:
1. copy or carefully remove this page
2. fill out the information,
3. return to the address below.

ORDER INFORMATION

NAME _____

STREET _____

CITY _____ STATE _____ ZIP _____

TOTAL BOOKS WANTED _____ @ 29.95 EACH _____
Indiana residents only add 5% sales tax. _____ @ 1.50 EACH _____
SHIPPING AND HANDLING _____ @ 5.00 EACH _____

TOTAL _____

CREDIT CARD ORDERS:

VISA ___ MASTERCARD ___ EXPIRATION DATE ____ / ____

NUMBER __ __ __ __ - __ __ __ __ - __ __ __ __ - __ __ __ __

SIGNATURE _____

SEND: TO:
1. This completed form   CERF (ACVO BOOK)
2. Check, money order (US funds)   1235 SCC-A
   OR include credit card information   Purdue University
                         W. Lafayette, IN 47907-1235